PRAISE FOR *AFTER ANY DIAGNOSIS*

"*After Any Diagnosis* should be a must for anyone who is managing a chronic disease or who has a life-threatening disease."

> NANCY DICKEY, M.D., Past President, American Medical Association; Interim Dean, Texas A&M University System College of Medicine

"Carol Svec has written an excellent book, which carefully and critically discusses important issues surrounding serious medical illness. I highly recommend it for patients and families facing difficult health problems."

> MAURIE MARKMAN, M.D., Director, The Cleveland Clinic Taussig Cancer Center; Chairman, Department of Hematology/Medical Oncology; The Lee and Jerome Burkons Research Chair in Oncology, The Cleveland Clinic Foundation, Cleveland, Ohio

"With its maze of diagnostic tests, technical jargon, and confusing treatment options, entering the health care system as a patient is like going to a foreign country where you don't speak the language. *After Any Diagnosis* is an absolutely essential resource to help you develop a road map to recovery. This book will empower you as a patient to become an active participant in overcoming your illness. Read this book, use it, and get better."

> WILLIAM W. DEARDOFF, PH.D., ABPP; Fellow, American Psychological Association; Diplomate, American Board of Clinical Health Psychology; Assistant Clinical Professor, UCLA School of Medicine; Coauthor of *Preparing for Surgery: A Mind-Body Approach to Enhance Healing and Recovery, Back Pain Remedies for Dummies,* and *Win the Battle Against Back Pain.*

"This book is well written and provides an excellent guide for a patient or family member to use when facing a long illness ahead. The intent of this guidebook is to empower the patient with information that is organized, concise, and clear, so he/she can make informed decisions about care as well as feel confident in the decisions being made on his/her behalf. Today, more than ever, patients need to take charge of their health. This book will help to achieve that end."

"Carol Svec's efforts at helping patients to become more knowledgeable, more insightful, and more involved in their care is valuable indeed."

"This is a very interesting and useful book which provides excellent data for people who are seriously researching their health problems. I believe that people who do have serious illness or unusual illness will be led to find legitimate information by the use of this book."

"*After Any Diagnosis* is a must read for anyone who has attempted to navigate the bewildering mass of medical information available. A well-informed patient is much more likely to comply with medical advice and do well, rather than simply endure treatment. Carol Svec provides an authoritative guide for seeking health information."

"This is an excellent book; a truly valuable and unique resource for any health-conscious consumer and an essential component to any personal library."

After Any Diagnosis

How to Take Action Against Your Illness Using the Best and Most Current Medical Information Available

CAROL SVEC

THREE RIVERS PRESS

NEW YORK

615.5071
5968

FOR BILL

for more reasons than I can name

This book is not intended as a substitute for the medical advice
of physicians. The reader should regularly consult his or her doctor
in matters relating to health.

Published by Three Rivers Press, New York, New York.
Member of the Crown Publishing Group.

Random House, Inc. New York, Toronto, London, Sydney, Auckland
www.randomhouse.com

THREE RIVERS PRESS is a registered trademark and the Three Rivers
Press colophon is a trademark of Random House, Inc.
Printed in the United States of America
Design by Susan Hood

Library of Congress Cataloging-in-Publication Data
Svec, Carol.
    After any diagnosis : how to take action against your illness using the
best and most current medical information available / Carol Svec.—1st ed.
    p. cm.
    1. Patient participation 2. Therapeutics—Decision making. I. Title.
R118.S87 2001
615.5'071—dc21   00-067303
ISBN 0-609-80669-6

10 9 8 7 6 5 4 3 2 1

First Edition

Acknowledgments

Most important, I need to thank the physicians, academics, and other health experts who voluntarily shared so much of their time and knowledge with me. Their high levels of enthusiasm, warmth, compassion, interest, and intelligence have been inspirational. I am honored to have had the chance to speak with such caring professionals as these.

Michael J. Barry, M.D.
  Chief of the General Medicine Unit, Massachusetts General Hospital
John D. Birkmeyer, M.D.
  Assistant professor of surgery, Dartmouth Medical School
Donald J. Cegala, Ph.D.
  Professor of Communication and Family Medicine, Ohio State University
Mary Jo Deering, Ph.D.
  Director of Health Communication and Telehealth for the Office of Disease Prevention and Health Promotion, U.S. Department of Health and Human Services
William C. Dooley, M.D.
  Director, Johns Hopkins Breast Center; chief of breast surgery, Johns Hopkins Hospital

Judith A. Erlen, Ph.D., R.N.
Professor and associate director of the Center for Research and
Chronic Disorders, University of Pittsburgh School of Nursing

Gary S. Francis, M.D.
Director, Coronary & Intensive Care Unit in Department of
Cardiology, Cleveland Clinic Foundation

Sheldon Greenfield, M.D.
Professor of medicine, Tufts University School of Medicine;
director, Primary Care Outcomes Research Institute,
New England Medical Center

Valerie Gross, M.L.S.
Community Health Resource Library librarian, Geisinger
Medical Center

John V. Guiliana, D.P.M.
Podiatrist, Hackettstown, New Jersey; educator in doctor-patient
communication

Vicki Helgeson, Ph.D.
Associate professor of psychology, Carnegie Mellon University

William T. Jarvis, Ph.D.
Professor of public health and preventive medicine,
Loma Linda University

Robert M. Kaplan, Ph.D.
Professor and chair of the Department of Family and Preventive
Medicine, University of California, San Diego

Sherrie H. Kaplan, Ph.D., M.P.H.
Associate professor of medicine at Tufts University School of
Medicine; codirector of the Primary Care Outcomes Research
Institute, New England Medical Center

Linda Farris Kurtz, D.P.A.
Professor in the Department of Social Work,
Eastern Michigan University

Forrest Lang, M.D.
Professor in the Department of Family Medicine, James H.
Quillen College of Medicine, East Tennessee State University

Susan Love, M.D.
Director, Susan Love Breast Cancer Foundation; founder,
SusanLoveMD.com; author of Dr. Susan Love's Breast Book

and Dr. Susan Love's Hormone Book; *adjunct professor of surgery at UCLA*

Maurie Markman, M.D.
Director, Cleveland Clinic Taussig Cancer Center

Dennis J. Mazur, M.D., Ph.D.
Professor of medicine, Oregon Health Sciences University; chairman, Institutional Review Board, Department of Veterans Affairs Medical Center, Portland, Oregon

Timothy B. McCall, M.D.
Internist; author of Examining Your Doctor: A Patient's Guide to Avoiding Harmful Medical Care; *founder, www.DrMcCall.com*

Neil B. Mehta, M.D.
Associate staff, Center for Medical Education, Research and Development, Department of General Internal Medicine, Cleveland Clinic Foundation

Stephen T. Mennemeyer, Ph.D.
Associate professor, School of Public Health, University of Alabama at Birmingham

Sheryl Merkin, M.S., R.N., C.D.E., C.P.T.
Diabetes clinical nurse specialist, Montefiore Medical Center

James M. Metz, M.D.
Assistant professor of radiation oncology, University of Pennsylvania; associate editor of the cancer website OncoLink

Annette O'Connor, R.N., Ph.D.
Professor, University of Ottawa School of Nursing and Faculty of Medicine; senior investigator, Ottawa Hospital Loeb Health Research Institute

Daniel O'Connor, Ph.D., M.L.S.
Associate professor, Department of Library and Information Science, Rutgers University

Michael J. Olek, M.D.
Clinical instructor, Harvard Medical School; attending physician, Brigham and Women's Hospital and Massachusetts General Hospital

Richard H. Price, D.M.D.
Spokesperson for American Dental Association; on staff at Boston University Dental School

Elaena Quattrocchi, B.S., Pharm. D., FASHP
  *Associate professor, pharmacy practice at Arnold and Marie
  Schwartz College of Pharmacy*
Robert G. Root, Ph.D.
  Associate professor, Department of Mathematics, Lafayette College
Ethan Russo, M.D.
  *Clinical assistant professor, Department of Medicine, University
  of Washington School of Medicine; board-certified child and adult
  neurologist, Montana Neurobehavioral Specialists*
Barbara Sanders, Ph.D., P.T., S.C.S.
  *Chair of the Department of Physical Therapy, Southwest Texas
  State University*
Lillie Shockney, R.N., B.S., M.A.S.
  Director of education and outreach, Johns Hopkins Breast Center

A few of these professionals deserve special thanks: Dr. Dennis
J. Mazur, for providing guidance and suggestions on the decision-
making chapter, above and beyond anything I could have
hoped for; Dr. Robert Root, for contributing substantially to
the chapter on statistics, making it much more thorough and
understandable; and Dr. John D. Birkmeyer, Dr. Donald J.
Cegala, Dr. Mary Jo Deering, Dr. Judith A. Erlen, Ms. Valerie
Gross, Dr. Vicki Helgeson, Dr. William T. Jarvis, Dr. Maurie
Markman, Dr. Richard H. Price, Dr. Elaena Quattrocchi, Dr.
Barbara Sanders, and Ms. Lillie Shockney, for reviewing earlier
versions of various chapters.

I also would like to give special thanks to the patients who
shared their stories with me in the hopes that others would
benefit from their experiences. Although in most cases their
names have been changed here, their tales are true and their
desire to help is heartfelt. I wish them the best of health.

I OWE A TREMENDOUS DEBT OF GRATITUDE to the people who
helped me take a concept and turn it into this book. My agent,
Jo Fagan of Jane Dystel Literary Management, gave this book
life by not throwing the proposal back in the slush pile. Plus,
she gives great advice. (And, Jane, thank you, too.) Peter Guz-

zardi, a genuinely warm and thoughtful person, first championed this book and made it a reality. My editor, Carrie Thornton, is always positive and encouraging, and makes the process seem easier than it is. I thank her for picking up an orphaned project and believing in my mission. Three Rivers Press executive editor Becky Cabaza took the extra effort to call and calm my skittish nerves during a critical time. She'll never know exactly how much that meant. And thanks to all the other talented people at Three Rivers—designers, copy editors, production managers, marketing and publicity folks, assistants, and executives. Every piece of the publishing puzzle is critical, and I applaud you all.

A<small>ND FINALLY,</small> THANK YOU TO:

Sid Kirchheimer, an amazing editor and friend, who got me my first freelance gig and taught me that no question should go unasked.

All the other amazing consumer health writers and editors I've worked with over the years, in particular: Michael Leff, who took "Lucy & Ethel" teamwork to a new level; Jeff Bredenberg, whose unwavering support was always appreciated; and David Freeman, who gave me a chance when he didn't have to.

The facilitators who helped me contact some of the health professionals interviewed for this book, especially Gary Stephenson of Johns Hopkins; Scott Tennant and Drez Jennings of the Cleveland Clinic; and Joel P. Smith, public affairs officer for the Portland, Oregon, VA Medical Center.

Dr. Christine Ganitsch, who is a perfect example of what a "good" doctor should be. Everyone should be so lucky as to have a doctor like her.

Henry Holland and Dolly Cinquino, excellent teachers from my formative years way back at "Cavallini." You two set me on the path of loving science and writing, so this is all your fault.

All my friends and family who encouraged and helped along the way, especially Wendy Potkay, Gene Potkay, Kristine Nelson, Brian Nelson, and Lois Hazel, who gave early suggestions about the book; the "Babes of Byron" (plus Kyle), whose enthusiasm kept me going; and Amanda and Kimberly Svec, who were always infectiously excited.

Teresa Lawrence and Ann Agrawal, for always being there. At all hours. Any time.

Ted Rudisill for offering a safety net I could never accept (but was comforted to have). Bill and Ginny Svec, Bob and Flo Svec, and Laura and Bill D'Addato, for always asking about the book, even when there were more important things to worry about. Bobby, Danny, Allison, Pamela, Asha, Alea, Megan, and Michael—just because.

And last, but never least, Marina Rudisill, who has been telling me for years that I should write a book. Mom, you're the best.

Contents

SECTION 1

Getting It Right from the Beginning

Introduction

GETTING diagnosed with an illness is like hearing the starting pistol at the beginning of a race. Whether it's a sprint or a marathon, a grueling endurance run or a jog through the park, the race is yours alone. No one can run it for you. And standing still is not an option—chances are the disease will progress if you don't take steps to halt it.

This book was written to help you run a better race, no matter what your diagnosis is, how old you are, or how long you've been ill.

When it comes to health care, we all want pretty much the same things: caring and competent doctors, effective treatments, and quality of life. The good news is that these things are more available now than ever before. The bad news is that you'll have to work to get them, but the results are well worth it.

The Good News

Despite the current fashion of portraying doctors as cold-hearted, money-hungry medicine machines, the truth is that the vast majority of doctors care deeply about the welfare of their patients. They can recall in specific detail those patients who presented the greatest challenge, or who overcame great odds, or whose illness somehow taught them to be better doctors. They feel the decline and deaths of their patients personally, and they hate when disease "wins." Even research doctors who never see patients because they spend their lives working in laboratories talk in idealistic terms of "finding a cure" or "making a contribution to humanity."

Forget about making money as a reason for becoming a doctor. Medicine is no longer a guaranteed lucrative profession. Doctors today must contend with the financial costs of medical school and malpractice insurance, and the realities of working in a managed care environment. It's been estimated that primary care physicians participating in managed care systems or HMOs need to see four patients per hour just to break even. This doesn't even take into account the personal costs of being on-call or working night shifts in a hospital, and the spiritual costs of having to tussle with insurance companies over appropriate care and coverage.

So why do they do it? The latest survey conducted by the Association of American Medical Colleges found that nearly 90 percent of students applying to medical school cited "making a difference in people's lives" as a very important reason for their career choice. "Prestige" and "high income" were far down the list, below "intellectual challenge" and "social responsibility."

As for treatments, there are now more options than ever for diagnosing, treating, and managing most diseases. The past few decades have brought about a tremendous expansion of medical knowledge and technology. For example, through telemedicine, doctors can communicate with each other via the Internet and telecommunication technologies nearly instantaneously across the globe. This means that doctors and patients in remote locations can benefit from the advice and consultation of the world's best specialists.

And many of the devices we take for granted today were mere science fiction just a generation or two ago. Ultrasound, now a part of routine prenatal care, wasn't used for medical purposes until the 1950s; now-familiar CAT scans and MRIs were only developed in the 1970s; and as this book is being written, scientists at the Johns Hopkins University School of Medicine are conducting tests to see if a laser-powered microchip implanted in the retina of the eye might help some blind people regain a portion of their sight. So much progress has been made in preventing, diagnosing, and treating some types of cancer that the death rate from cancer has declined for the first time since the 1930s.

Quality of life is also more easily attainable these days. In the past several years, the medical community has been reevaluating the role of medications in pain control, placing more emphasis on relieving a patient's discomfort than on the possibility of drug dependence or side effects. Doctors have also begun fostering partner relationships with their patients, as opposed to the traditional paternalistic model of treatment. Time and again, studies have shown that patients feel greater satisfaction and are more likely to comply with their treatment schedules when they are involved in their health care. Some studies have even shown that when patients are well-informed and participate in making medical decisions, their physical and psychological health improves. This information has not been lost on clinicians—dozens of medical schools in the United States currently have formalized doctor-patient communication programs, and more will undoubtedly follow.

The Bad News

I hate to be the one to break it to you, but the days of the all-knowing Marcus Welby–like family physician are over (if they ever actually existed). The most well-intentioned physician is constrained by managed care rules, which usually means seeing more patients for shorter amounts of time. According to a study published in 1999 by researchers from Harvard Medical School, Johns Hopkins University, and other institutions, the average office visit lasts approximately eighteen minutes. In that time the doctor needs to greet the patient, review the patient's chart, talk about the reason for the current visit, conduct a physical examination, write notes in the chart, answer questions, and give medication or treatment instructions. That doesn't leave much time for hand-holding or empathizing with the patient, and so doctors appear cold and uncaring.

Plus, we can no longer simply trust that our primary care physician will know the latest treatments. There is so much new information generated that no one doctor can keep track of it all. Every year more than 4,000 biomedical journals are published, and the FDA approves about 550 drugs for new or expanded use and about 3,700 new medical devices. State-of-the-art treatments may go untried simply because your doctor hasn't had time to read about them yet. In a study published in the *New England Journal of Medicine*, one-in-four primary care physicians surveyed said they worried that the scope of care they were expected to provide was too large, and would be better handled by specialists. And yet the managed care system dictates that they continue to treat these more difficult cases. If doctors themselves don't feel confident of their abilities, how can we be expected to entrust our health to them?

More devastating can be medical mistakes. Moving more and more patients through physicians' offices in less and less time not only hurts the doctor-patient relationship, some experts say it compromises the quality of care and may increase the chance that a mistake will be made. According to a controversial 1999 report by the Institute of Medicine, between 44,000 and 98,000 deaths are caused by medical mistakes each year, prompting hospitals, organizations, and government committees to look for ways to reduce the errors. Until then, patients need to find out how they can protect themselves.

One small personal example: I was advised to have a contrast CAT scan to determine the cause of some recurring abdominal pain. When asked directly, my doctor and the CAT technician told me the procedure was perfectly safe. But being the obsessive health researcher that I am, I took one additional and very simple step that proved to be critical. I looked up "CAT scan" in a book of medical procedures. There was a warning in bold type saying that CAT contrast dyes contain iodine, which can cause a serious reaction in people who are allergic to shellfish. Guess what I'm allergic to! My doctor hadn't warned me, and the CAT technician only asked if I had an allergy to medications. If I hadn't bothered to check up on the procedure, a simple twenty-minute test could have landed me in the hospital . . . or even, depending on the severity of my allergic reaction, taken my life.

The lesson is this: If you want the best medical care . . . if you want to be able to take advantage of all the high-tech advances available . . . if you want a better chance of understanding and managing your disease, then you need to become more actively involved in your health care.

Think back to the last time you purchased a car. You probably did several things to make sure you made the best possible decision. You may have asked your friends how they liked their cars, looked in automotive or consumer magazines for the latest ratings, read newspaper articles, went to the showroom to test-drive the model you wanted, looked at other cars for comparison, and hunted around for the lowest price. We need to make at least that much of an effort when pursuing something even more precious—our health.

Why Read This Book

William C. Dooley, M.D., a surgical oncologist at Johns Hopkins Hospital and director of the Johns Hopkins Breast Center, once told me that the first thing he tells his newly diagnosed patients is to go out and gather as much information about their disease as they possibly can. After a pause, he sighed and said, "Unfortunately, very few people know how to do that."

This book was written to help you learn how to gather, understand, and use medical information. It is based on published research, interviews with top physicians and experts from across the country, patients' personal stories, and my own professional experience. As a health writer and researcher, I need to locate and digest information on a wide variety of medical topics quickly. The information has to be current and accurate, otherwise I'm out of a job. If you are dealing with an illness, the stakes are much higher for you. This book will guide you through the process of becoming a more active patient and, it is hoped, a healthier person.

Since everyone's needs are different, this book was designed to allow you to pick and choose the sections you want to focus on, in any order. I recommend that you read Section One, "Getting It Right from the Beginning," in its entirety first. It describes why learning more about your disease and doctor-patient partnering are important to your health, the type of information you need, how to start an information search, and how to organize the information you find.

Section Two, "Information Sources," talks about various information sources and how to use them to your best advantage: How accurate is the health information in books, newsletters, and newspaper articles? Where is the best information on the Internet? How can you tell the difference between a "good" source and one that may be misleading or wrong? How can you access and start to understand the same sources of medical information your doctor uses? The sources are rated for accessibility and usefulness, and a summary is included at the end of each chapter for easy reference.

Section Three, "Caregivers," discusses how to find the best medical care by researching doctors, hospitals, other caregivers, and support groups: How can you find the best doctor for you? Are some hospitals better than others? What other health specialists should you tap for information? Are all support groups the same?

Section Four, "Putting It All Together," describes how to use the information you've gathered, including a brief and painless (I hope) chapter on statistics to help you understand some of the numbers you read, and a chapter on the nuts and bolts of making a medical decision.

This book is not intended to help you diagnose an illness—no book can do that. Nor does this book advocate alternative treatments over standard medicine. The information-gathering skills that are covered here are designed to help you become a better health partner with your doctor so that the two of you, together, can treat and manage your illness. Physicians, medical technology, and scientific methods still offer the best options for cure, recovery, and life extension.

Treat this book as you would a cookbook, as a basic set of instructions that can be adapted to include your own innovations and style as you become more comfortable with information gathering. Once you have the skills, you'll develop your own shortcuts and favorite resources to which you can return as you manage your illness throughout the years.

Like all families, mine has been hit by quite a few illnesses over the years, some serious, some not so serious. Time and time again, my familiarity with research has allowed me to interpret medical information for people I love. What I've discovered is that different people use the information in different ways. Some use it as a way to understand and gain control over their fears and anxiety. Others use it as a tool to seek out the best care. Still others use large quantities of information to guide their decision making. Since everyone is different, all these responses are "right" for the particular individual involved.

A few years ago, my youngest sister was diagnosed with a brain tumor the size of an orange. I've never had such an electric jolt of fear as when I heard her tell me those words over the telephone. I spent the next twenty-four hours straight finding all the information I could about her type of tumor (a meningioma) and calling other family members to tell them what I had been able to learn. Because the tumor was benign, the information was generally a comfort. But because of the large size of the tumor, the surgery would be tricky. We found out there was a chance of paralysis, brain damage, and loss of memory. Over the next couple of weeks, as she prepared for surgery, more research told us that her doctor was among the best in the country, that the hospital had state-of-the-art technology for brain surgery, and what to expect during recovery. Although we couldn't take away the reality of the disease, we could understand it and prepare for all potential outcomes. Fortunately, my sister was treated well, and the biggest remnant of the ordeal is a four-inch-square scar that shows where titanium plates hold the pieces of her skull together. (I think it is a tribute to her resilience that she likes to show it off at parties!)

With each diagnosis—from my sister's brain tumor to my brother-in-law's avascular necrosis and hip replacement to a friend's thyroid cancer and other illnesses of friends and family—I've been fortunate enough to be able to help by providing information and talking them (and their families) through the treatment and healing process. It is my sincere wish that this book accomplish the same for you by providing a place to start in understanding and managing your illness.

1. Information—Why Bother?

IMAGINE undergoing surgery, taking large amounts of medications that cause you to feel even sicker than you already do, suffering nearly unendurable pain, and perhaps dying . . . without ever knowing why.

That scenario is unthinkable in the United States. But in many cultures today, a majority of doctors report that they don't tell patients about their disease if the diagnosis is cancer. They tell the families, and the families make medical decisions without ever telling the patient what is wrong. Patients who suspect cancer and directly ask their doctors about it are often lied to. Although the diagnosis is withheld out of compassion, to save the patient from worry, it seems cruel and unethical to current Western sensibilities.

That example seems so extreme that it might surprise you to hear that until about thirty years ago many doctors in the United States had the same nondisclosure policy. Fortunately, that particular practice has changed, but other forms of information are still being withheld:

- In 1999, researchers at Northwestern University found that many women in the United States who had had a breast removed to treat breast cancer (mastectomy) *had not been told* that there was another treatment just as effective that would spare the breast (lumpectomy with radiation).

- Many men who undergo treatment for prostate cancer *are not told* in advance that two common side effects are impotence and urinary incontinence.
- Despite the fact that statin drugs significantly reduce cholesterol levels, can decrease the risk of heart attack by about one-third, and have virtually no side effects, many at-risk patients *are not told* that this treatment option exists.

These are just some examples, but similar stories can be found for just about any disease or condition. Why the secrecy? It's not that these tight-lipped physicians are incompetent, or that they are deliberately trying to torture us or keep us ill. These types of problems stem from three main roots.

First, there are time constraints for talking with patients. The average office visit rarely lasts more than sixteen minutes. In that time, doctors feel lucky if they can communicate one or two main pieces of information. Given the choice of spending that time explaining the benefits of diet and exercise for controlling cholesterol, for example, or launching into a full explanation of statin drugs, some doctors choose to focus on the drugs. Doctors tend to be more familiar with drugs than nutrition, and a pill is easier to prescribe than a diet. And if the patient has more than one problem, say diabetes and high cholesterol, the physician is more likely to focus on the immediate problem of controlling blood sugar than on the more subtle problem of lowering cholesterol.

"I think most doctors would say that lack of time really is a problem for patient education in general, and for shared decision making in particular," says Michael J. Barry, M.D., chief of the General Medicine Unit at Massachusetts General Hospital in Boston. "Every doctor I know feels pressed to see more patients in the same amount of time. That squeezes what needs to be done. And frankly, for more complicated medical problems, [it] may squeeze out time to have a good medical conversation. Doctors may tell patients what to do just to move on more quickly."

Second, some doctors may not tell everything about a disease because they may not know the latest information, or they may be wary of anything new. New drugs, new procedures, and new studies continually change and challenge medicine's status quo. Some doctors (like many of the rest of us) are slow to incorporate new ideas into their daily practices. But even the best-intentioned doctors find there simply is not enough time to keep up with the onslaught of information. For example, patients may not be told that breast-sparing surgery is often just as effective as mastectomy in some cases either because their doctors haven't kept up with the science or because they'd rather continue to perform the surgery they are most familiar with, the mastectomy.

Third, information transfer may be limited because many doctors still believe in the old-fashioned, physician-focused mode of communication called paternalism. In a stereotypical paternal relationship, the physician acts toward patients as a father acts toward small children. The physician is believed to be all-knowing and directs patients toward what the physician thinks is the best disease treatment. On the other hand, the patient is believed to be emotional and ignorant about medical issues.

A paternalistic relationship with your doctor requires blind trust in the physician—after all, father knows best. For this reason, a patient's feelings and desires about medical treatment are discounted as unimportant to the process. Very little explanation of the disease, medication, or treatment is given to the patient because, well, it would be just too much for our "child-like" little heads to absorb and understand, and we are expected to comply without question or complaint.

I heard a frightening example of paternalism when I spoke with Loretta. When Loretta felt a lump in her breast, she did what every woman is advised to do—she went to her physician to have it checked out. The doctor felt the lump and told her he thought it was benign. At age thirty-seven, Loretta was considered at low risk for cancer. The doctor sent her across the hall to a colleague, a general surgeon, who also believed the lump was benign. He ordered a mammogram and an ultra-sound, but never did a standard needle biopsy, in which a slen-der needle is guided into the breast to remove a tiny portion of the lump so the surgeon would know exactly what he was dealing with. Surgery was recommended to remove the lump, but no one thought it might be cancer. By the time the surgery was scheduled two months later, Loretta told her doctor that the lump had grown noticeably, but the surgeon told her that it was all in her imagination. He still was not concerned.

Under local anesthesia (which meant that Loretta was awake through the whole ordeal) in an out-patient facility, with no preoperative testing, the doctor sliced into her breast. What started out as a simple forty-five-minute procedure ended up taking a grueling one hour and forty-five minutes. The doctor took a biopsy, sent it to pathology, closed her wound, got a call from pathology, reopened her wound, and did more surgery. There was trouble. Not only was the lump malignant, but the incision went through the heart of the cancer and the sur-rounding blood vessels, spreading cancerous cells throughout her breast.

Up to that point, Loretta had been a passive patient who believed what her paternalistic doctor told her, just as many of us do. She trusted his opinion that the lump was not cancerous, and she trusted that he referred her to a competent surgeon. She trusted that the surgeon would do all the standard tests, and take all necessary precautions. She trusted that everything would be OK.

Hindsight is twenty-twenty, so there's a good chance many of us would have been just as trusting. How many times have you taken a prescription without really knowing what it was for, when to take it, or what the side effects might be? How many times have you accepted a diagnosis that didn't quite seem right, only to find out later that the diagnosis was wrong? This is the way most of us were taught to deal with doctors and illness. Granted, not all outcomes are as devastating as Loretta's, but that type of philosophy makes abuse or thoughtless adherence to a treatment pattern more likely.

Fortunately, many experts are predicting that, in the near future, paternalism will no longer be a viable model for doctors to follow. Demands of patients, greater access to health information, and the time-limiting realities of working under a managed care health system will require that a new type of relationship develop, one in which patients and physicians form a synergistic partnership that respects the intelligence, wisdom, and decision-making abilities on both sides of the diagnosis.

Medical Partnerships

The medical community has been researching and discussing the idea of patient participation for years, but only recently has discussion turned into active promotion. The World Health Organization has come out in favor of a patient's right to influence medical decisions, and the latest edition of the ethics manual of the American College of Physicians explicitly talks about doctor-patient relationships and a patient's right to informed consent. Some states have even passed legislation making physicians legally accountable for failing to disclose certain types of information to their patients. For example, at least eighteen states now require physicians to tell breast cancer patients all their treatment options.

Even the respected American Medical Association, previously thought to be a bastion of paternalism, is endorsing partnerships as beneficial to both doctors and patients. The organization has published patient-oriented guidelines on physician-patient partnerships.

In a medical partnership, the physician and the patient work together to decide the best treatment for that individual patient. Each side has something valuable to bring to the medical decision-making process: The physician offers years of medical education and treatment experience, and the patient brings his or her own life history, firsthand experience of symptoms, values, preferences, and goals. Only when both sides work together can the illness be treated in a manner most likely to promote physical healing without harming the patient or compromising his or her quality of life.

There are very few situations in which being active will not help. The only exceptions are dire emergencies, when there is no time to become involved. Otherwise, any time you have a chronic disease, use a medication, try alternative treatments, or see a physician, you have an opportunity to become active and involved. "The more active the patient is, the more likely their needs will get tended to," said Sheldon Greenfield, M.D., director of the Primary Care Outcomes Research Institute (PCORI) at the New England Medical Center and professor of medicine at Tufts University School of Medicine in Boston.

Being active is especially important when facing complex medical decisions. If the outcome of treatment is uncertain, or if the risks and benefits have the potential of having a great impact on the patient's life, the patient needs to be involved in the decision. For example, patient involvement is not critical for proper treatment of a simple throat infection—antibiotics will clear it up with no serious side effects. But what if a patient needs treatment for blocked arteries? The treatment decision is complex and may have serious outcomes. Follow this example:

Two possible treatments for widening blocked arteries are angioplasty and drugs. The decision is difficult. During angioplasty, a small tube is inserted into an artery in the groin, then carefully guided up to the blocked area near the heart. A small balloon is inflated, squeezing the fatty tissue against the artery wall and opening the pathway for the blood to flow. The procedure is successful 90 percent of the time, but blockage returns for about 40 percent of patients in six months. Further, a small number of patients die of a heart attack or blood clot during or soon after the procedure. Drugs unblock the arteries more slowly, but there is no risk of death. Both options seem to offer the same level of protection against future heart attack and death.

So the choices are (simplified here for this example): (a) a procedure that carries a small risk of immediate death, with benefits that may last only a few months but will reduce pain; or (b) drugs that won't reduce pain as well but will reduce long-term death rate to the same as angioplasty and won't cause immediate death. Would you want your doctor to choose for you? Or would you want to discuss all the risks, benefits, and possible outcomes before coming to an informed decision with the help of your doctor? If you chose the latter, you are ready to become an active patient. (Seems kind of obvious when presented that way, doesn't it?)

When asked, most people would prefer this type of participation, also known as "shared decision making." Those who want less responsibility tend to be sicker, older, or feel helpless about their condition, which is understandable because those patients will generally have less strength and energy to devote to being active, and the elderly usually have decades of experience surviving under paternal care. Most patients, however, want as much information as possible. To illustrate, researchers at Albany Medical College in New York found that 92 percent of cancer patients they interviewed wanted to hear all the information about their disease, regardless of whether it was good or bad news. (Not receiving information commonly leads to frustration, anxiety, and/or anger.)

Aside from merely feeling more involved, active patients are physically and emotionally better off than more passive patients. Over the past twenty-five years, research has shown that patients who participate are generally more satisfied with their health care, have a better understanding of their illness, cope with their disease better, are less anxious before medical procedures, comply with treatments more fully, are hospitalized less frequently, and claim to have a better quality of life. "The more patients know," says Gary Francis, M.D., director of the Coronary Intensive Care Unit at the Cleveland Clinic Foundation, "the better informed they are, the more likely they are to keep their appointments, to take their medications, to stay on their specialized diets."

Some doctors believe that informed patients may be more likely to seek and receive the best care. "Patients who are more active in understanding their disease tend to do better in general," says William C. Dooley, M.D., director of the Johns Hopkins Breast Center. "These patients will generally know very quickly if they are being sold a false bill of goods, whereas patients who haven't invested much time in learning about their disease may go along with [treatments] which may not even make good common sense, much less medical sense."

As if that weren't enough, active patients tend to get better faster and maintain better health. According to Sherrie Kaplan, Ph.D., M.P.H., associate professor of medicine at Tufts University School of Medicine in Boston and one of the leading researchers in the area of patient participation, active patients don't just say they feel better, they have actual, measurable health improvements. Studies have shown that patients who are more involved, who ask more questions, and try to direct the flow of conversation during an office visit lose fewer days of work due to their illness. Active patients with diabetes maintain better control of their disease, as measured by lower blood sugar; and active patients with hypertension maintain lower blood pressure readings than passive patients. Other studies have found that active patients with cancer experience fewer chemotherapy symptoms, are less depressed, report lower levels of pain, and maintain better physical and emotional functioning compared with more passive patients. And active patients even recover faster after surgery, leading to a quicker release from the hospital.

Physicians have been slow to adopt medical partnerships with their patients. A study published in the January 2000 issue of the *Journal of the American Medical Association* found that patients were fully informed in only 9 percent of 3,552 medical decisions monitored during the research. In general, there was little or no discussion of the uncertainties involved with the decisions, patient preferences, or patient understanding.

Given how much physicians have to gain from patient partnerships, the reluctance to involve patients seems all the more puzzling. All physicians are under the gun to give patients more information in order to comply with informed consent laws. And if patients are well informed and prepared to discuss their medical conditions and treatment, it can take a big burden off physicians' shoulders, according to Robert Kaplan, Ph.D., professor and chair of the Department of Family and Preventive Medicine at the University of California, San Diego. "I think a lot of practitioners feel awkward being confronted with a complicated question, realizing they don't have time to deal with it," he says.

An informed patient allows doctors to focus on specific issues and treatment, instead of spending precious time explaining disease basics. "It doesn't make a lot of sense for me as a physician to explain to a patient, say, what a prostate is and what it does. That can easily be done by someone else or some other materials," says Dr. Michael Barry. "What I like to do is educate [patients] to a certain level using those other resources, and then try to use my time to match their preferences with the treatments."

"Many physicians really do appreciate patients who are organized, who can present a complete history, who bring copies of test results or procedures, who do ask questions when they're confused about matters and so on," says Donald J. Cegala, Ph.D., professor of communication and family medicine at Ohio State University. "Of course, physicians are people, and there are going to be differences among physicians and some probably are going to be even irritated at patients' questions. But from my experience, and with the majority of physicians I have seen and talked with, they are much more positive than negative about this sort of [partnership]."

"Doctors love those kinds of patients," agrees Dr. Sheldon Greenfield. For doctors who aren't engaging in these kinds of partnership relationships now, the good news is patients can push them or encourage them to do it. "If the patient is active and handles the doctor correctly, most doctors will be very pleased to go along," Dr. Greenfield notes. Occasionally you may find a doctor who is totally unresponsive and unwilling to form an active partnership. In that case, follow Dr. Greenfield's advice and "leave the doctor." After all, your health depends on it.

Oh, and remember Loretta? Her story didn't end the day of what she calls her "doomsday" breast surgery. That very day, she took control and became an active patient.

2. Becoming an Active Patient

IT was like a shockwave hit me. . . . All I could think was, 'I've got cancer. I'm going to die,'" says Loretta of her ordeal in 1997. Things got worse before they got better. She wouldn't be alive today if not for her fighting spirit and her decision to become an active patient, which included seeking out the best medical care possible and being a part of every treatment decision.

"That day I was diagnosed, I called my sister-in-law, a nurse, and I told her I had cancer. She said, 'You come down here.' So we drove down to North Carolina with my son that night. By the time we got down there, my sister had already started gathering information for me from Internet sources. I was scared that everything I would learn I wouldn't want to know. And there was so much I didn't know.

"Initially, what I started learning when I got on the Internet was creating a lot of anxiety because it was information that wasn't making sense to me. At that time, I thought I had a two-centimeter lump. So I looked that up and said, 'Oh good, I'm only at Stage Two.' But then, do I have metastases . . . what's that? Lymph nodes . . . what are you talking about? Axillary node dissection . . . what? What? What? I was trying to take on the stress of the new diagnosis, along with trying to gather new information. I didn't even give myself a chance to breathe, to make it all make sense.

"Over that first weekend, my sister-in-law and my family were a big comfort to me. My sister took me to the bookstore and bought me *Dr. Susan Love's Breast Book* as a gift. I didn't know what it was at the time, but it jumped out as probably one of the better books to have, because when we flipped through it, it seemed to cover a lot of good stuff. It's one of my prized possessions. It gave me enough of an understanding and answers to certain questions so that when I would wake up at three o'clock in the morning and say, 'Oh my gosh, I've got to know the answer to this,' it gave me some level of comfort."

Five days after arriving at her sister-in-law's, Loretta got an appointment at one of the premier breast treatment centers in the United States. And during the next year, she had a mastectomy, chemotherapy, a bone marrow transplant, and radiation, followed by delayed reconstruction of the breast. At each step she continued reading, researching, learning, and taking charge of her treatments. As of this writing, she has no remaining cancer in her body. Her doctors and nurses say her active involvement contributed greatly to her recovery.

According to Sherrie Kaplan, Ph.D., M.P.H., associate professor of medicine at Tufts University School of Medicine and codirector of the Primary Care Outcome Research Institute at the New England Medical Center in Boston, the lifetime probability of being a patient in the United States is virtually 100 percent. In contrast, the lifetime probability of being in a house fire is exceedingly small. Yet we spend more public and private resources on telling people how to get out of a burning house than we do on telling them how to be an effective patient. "Certainly, the one arena where we could make a big difference is teaching people from childhood how to be more involved in their health care," says Dr. Sherrie Kaplan. That type of training has the potential to save more lives than all the fire drills you can hold.

The basics of how to be an active patient can be learned relatively easily. The American Academy on Physician and Patient distributes a one-page flyer explaining how patients can become more involved in their medical care. Donald J. Cegala, Ph.D., professor of communication and family medicine at Ohio State University, has found that a fourteen-page take-home training booklet provides enough information to help patients ask questions, express concerns, and verify their understanding during an office visit. And Dr. Sherrie Kaplan and her colleagues at the New England Medical Center have developed a more involved twenty-minute, one-on-one training session. She and Dr. Sheldon Greenfield are even training children with chronic illnesses how to become active patients with the help of interactive videos and a board game.

But learning the skills and putting them to use in front of a doctor are two very different things. Any medical visit is an anxiety-producing situation, which makes practicing active patient skills next to impossible. "That people manage to do it at all is a wonderment," says Dr. Sherrie Kaplan. "Nervous and naked is how you usually are in a doctor's examining room. Imagine taking a math test nervous and naked. How would you do?"

What typically happens is that you're sitting in the examining room with questions to ask, but in the stress and rush of the moment you've forgotten what they are. If you're managing a chronic disease, the next time you're going to see this physician is probably three to six months later. So you have an eighteen-minute session with the doctor, and then you've got to take over and manage your own condition. On top of that, the doctor rushes through explanations, and may forget to tell you a fact or two. Unless you are prepared in advance, chances are very small that you'll leave the office knowledgeable, satisfied, and well-prepared to take care of your illness.

▶ ACTION PLAN

These action points outline the basics of what it takes to be an active patient, and provide tips for incorporating these new skills into your next office visit. As with all skills, there are multiple levels of difficulty and sophistication. Becoming proficient will take time, but you can do it. The biggest requirement is a desire to gain control over your illness.

Most of the real work comes up front, when you'll have to spend time seeking out information and learning about your disease and its treatment. Rather than being tedious, most patients find this process energizing and encouraging. One patient interviewed even said he felt it was like being on a treasure hunt, looking for a way to get better faster. Loretta claims that doing the research helped calm her down when she was most nervous about her prospects as a breast cancer patient by making her feel she was doing something productive.

Read through all the action items, then choose one or two you'd like to start with. Work with those until you feel comfortable, then add a couple more to your skill base. You'll probably find that certain actions will become second nature very quickly, while others may take a while to get used to. Don't get discouraged. After all, you're bucking a lifetime of health care habits. Although these strategies are considered optimal by people who study doctor-patient relationships, you may find that you can obtain the same results by modifying them to fit your personality. (For example, if you are extremely shy and unwilling to ask questions in person, you may be able to e-mail questions to your doctor.) But whatever you do, don't expect perfection—even people who work in this field admit that they sometimes fall back into old patterns and habits. Consider it a lifetime project dedicated to your health.

▶ ACTION ITEM 1: *Seek out and understand information about your disease and treatment.*
This is the foundation upon which all other action points rest. If you understand what your disease is, what may have caused it, what makes it worse, what makes it better, what is typical, and what might be unusual, you will be able to monitor your health better. You'll know what to expect in the future. You'll

know when something is wrong and when to see the doctor. You'll be aware of new treatments that might be better than what you are currently doing.

How much information do you really need? According to nearly every doctor interviewed for this book, there is no such thing as too much information. Knock yourself out. Gather as much information as you feel capable of handling, then go back for more once you've had a chance to review and understand it all.

"One of the arguments that people make is that you shouldn't [gather medical information] because people are overwhelmed and confused and it causes anxiety. . . . I don't believe that's so," says Robert Kaplan, Ph.D., professor and chair of the Department of Family and Preventive Medicine at the University of California, San Diego. In his research he found that while there may be some initial anxiety, over the long run patients almost always feel better when they have information and participate in shared decision making.

Traditional thinking was that there were different types of people who did better with different amounts of information. The theory was that people who love detail and want to hear every scrap of information do best when their needs are met, whereas those who prefer to stay in the dark do better if kept in the dark. The most recent research does not support that hypothesis. In a majority of studies, passive, uninformed patients were more depressed, functioned less well, had poorer quality of life, managed their diseases more poorly, and recovered less quickly than active patients.

How to find and understand information is what the rest of this book is about.

▶ ACTION ITEM 2: *Establish partnerships with your doctors.*

Before you can form a good working partnership with your doctor, you must first conquer your fear of physicians. Realize that they are human beings who just happen to have had a lot of education that gave them medical knowledge you can tap into. They are not saviors (although certain television dramas portray them to be), and they are not perfect. Of course, when you are very sick, it's easy to believe that your physician holds the power of life and death. That's enough to make anyone fearful of questioning, contradicting, or offending. Work to get over that feeling by telling your doctor how you feel, and that you'd like to develop a more comfortable working relationship. Once these fears are out in the open, they often lessen and disappear with time. The truth is that you have the best chance for getting top-notch medical care when you and your doctor work together to solve your health problem.

Talk to your doctor about wanting to participate more fully in decisions, and make him or her aware of the steps you are taking to find out more about your condition. If necessary, make a separate appointment to do this, and ask to have the discussion in the office, not the examining room. A less clinical environment will help you feel more comfortable.

Be direct when approaching your doctor about becoming a medical partner, suggests Forrest Lang, M.D., professor in the Department of Family Medicine at James H. Quillen College of Medicine at East Tennessee State University. Ask the physician directly. Your doctor may even beat you to the punch. Current recommendations are for physicians to take the initiative and explore the degree to which patients want to be active partners in decision making.

After you get over the initial hurdle, talk with your doctor about your mutual expectations from this new partnership. After that, the goal is to find ways to work together. What you are looking for is "common ground," a term Dr. Lang uses when he teaches physicians and medical students about doctor-patient partnerships. "When you start to look at it, there are differences of expectation in 30 to 50 percent of visits," says Dr. Lang. The patient goes to the doctor expecting something specific—a shot of penicillin, a prescription for a narcotic, a referral for an MRI. On the other hand, the physician may feel that these are not the appropriate interventions at that point. In that situation, the patient and the physician are not on common ground. The idea is to have each side listen to the expectations of the other, and work toward a solution that both are comfortable with.

Plan to keep the dialog about expectations going throughout the partnership. Your needs will change as you progress as an active patient. In the beginning, you may need to ask a few additional questions per session. Later, you may be bringing journal articles to discuss. Clarify protocol issues as they arise. For example, if you find yourself with a lot of questions between office visits, ask how you might get those questions answered. Some physicians prefer you to leave a phone message that they can have a nurse return later, others accept faxed or e-mailed questions, still others set aside time to respond to calls personally.

A word of caution: The sense of empowerment and control that many patients feel once they become more active can be exciting. Care has to be taken not to abuse this newfound sense of power. Don't be tempted to start making independent decisions about your health care, demanding certain medications or procedures, or monopolizing your doctor's time. The trick is to prepare for the office visit (see Action Item 6) so thoroughly that you can get the information you need within the usual amount of time and maintain a healthy partnership. If your doctor refuses to treat you as a partner or discourages questions, find a new doctor. Your doctor should be an ally, not an antagonist.

▶ ACTION ITEM 3: *Be entirely open with your physician.* Some patients expect their doctors to be mind readers. They don't mention a new symptom just to see if the doctor discovers it, or they figure that it's the doctor's job to ask all the right questions. A working doctor-patient partnership includes a two-way exchange of information. Share all your concerns, all your questions, and all your symptoms (even the embarrassing ones). If you've been under additional stress, if you've changed your diet or exercise routine, or traveled to a foreign country recently, let your doctor know. All these factors may affect your health. If your doctor says something that worries or offends you, mention it. If you think you have cancer, or you saw a television show that worried you, mention it.

"[Patients] tell us that they often feel foolish saying they think they have cancer," says Dr. Forrest Lang, "but how can you reach common ground, how can you negotiate what really can be done to alleviate your concerns unless you tell someone what your concerns are?" That's the only way you and your doctor can come up with an appropriate treatment plan. Plus, your openness is a signal to the doctor that he or she can be entirely open with you.

Being entirely open also means telling your doctor if you don't intend to follow treatment instructions. Don't just say what you think the doctor wants to hear. According to Sheldon Greenfield, M.D., director of the Primary Care Outcomes Research Institute (PCORI) at the New England Medical Center and professor of medicine at Tufts University School of Medicine, most people leave the doctor's office saying "Yes, yes, yes" to everything the doctor says, but they have no intention of following through. "They don't see themselves as joining hands with the doctor in a treatment plan or diagnostic," says Dr. Greenfield. This only harms your health and can undermine your partnership status with your physician.

"If somebody is fully informed and makes an agreement, says that's what I'm going to do, the expectation is that they will follow through with that," says Dr. Lang. "If the patient becomes disenchanted or unhappy, most physicians would appreciate patients coming back and saying, 'I tried this and it didn't work,' or 'I tried this and I have some new concerns,' rather than going to someone else."

If you have concerns or a problem following a treatment plan, inform your doctor so you can work toward a solution together. For example, if you know that you never remember to take your medication, tell your doctor. He or she could tell you that there are new devices that sound an alert when it is time to take pills, or you may be able to get injections instead. Or, if swallowing pills is the problem, perhaps there's a liquid form of the medication that would go down easier. Or, if there are too many side effects, your doctor may be able to change medications or reassure you that those side effects will disappear in a week. For any treatment option, if you haven't been able to follow the doctor's recommendation, discuss it. You'll feel better for not having to sneak around and for communicating your fears, and you and your doctor can find a better treatment.

▶ ACTION ITEM 4: *Don't leave the office without understanding what your doctor said.*

Have you ever walked out of the doctor's office and asked yourself, "Now, what was I supposed to do again?" Most of us have. The best way to ensure that you understand what was said is to repeat the instructions back to your doctor. Listen all the way through, then say, "OK, here's what I understand I'm supposed to do. . . ." If you get something wrong, your doctor will tell you. Write down special instructions or things you want to remember immediately, instead of trusting your memory when you try to recall the information later.

Questioning always leads to better understanding. If you don't understand your diagnosis, treatment, or other explanation, keep asking questions until you get answers that mean something to you. If the answer is still confusing, ask again. And if you still don't understand after the third try, ask if there is a physician's assistant or nurse who might be able to explain it to you.

It is especially important to ask about new medications. What is the medication supposed to do? What are the potential side effects? Is there anything you should or shouldn't do when taking the medication (such as, don't drive or don't drink alcohol)? Will this conflict with any other medication you are currently taking? *(Always carry with you a list of the medications you are taking, including dosage and the number of times per day you take them.)* Keep it handy in your wallet or purse. Many times patients have several different prescriptions from different physicians. A single list will help each doctor understand the full scope of treatment, avoid duplicating a prescription, and ensure that potentially dangerous combinations of drugs are not given. In an emergency, this medications list will allow hospital personnel to treat you more quickly.

▶ ACTION ITEM 5: *Bring a friend.*

Another way to improve understanding is to bring a friend or family member with you to the office visit. Have that person in the room to hear everything the doctor says and, if possible, take notes. "Somebody else in the room makes the doctor speak to everybody, [makes the doctor] make sure everything's clear, make sure it's right, make sure it's understandable," says Dr. Sheldon Greenfield. Plus, you'll get more time. Research has shown that physicians spend more time with a patient when family members are present. Later, that person will make a good sounding board if you need to remember specific details or decide on a course of action.

Some doctors encourage their patients to bring a tape recorder to the office visit. This is especially helpful for frightening diseases, such as cancer, since high emotionality tends to limit our recall of facts. It is also very helpful in cases where the treatment options have complex sets of risks and benefits. Patients can listen to the tape as many times as necessary to clarify their understanding.

Many doctors don't allow tape recordings, mainly for fear that the tapes may come back to haunt them in future potential lawsuits. In reality, tape recordings can also work to protect doctors by proving that they fully informed their patients about medical procedures. If you feel strongly that you would like to record your sessions, speak honestly with your doctor about your need to hear the information more than once. If he or she still won't allow it, ask how else you might get the same information to review at home, or seek out a different doctor who will be more willing to work with you.

▶ ACTION ITEM 6: *Prepare for office visits.*

The key to a productive office visit is twofold: (1) understanding and preparing the kinds of information a physician is likely to need, and (2) organizing your questions. For both these areas, write down your thoughts in advance and bring your notes with you to the doctor. It's very easy to forget even critical pieces of information in the stress of an exam, so bring a detailed reminder list. If you copy and complete the Doctor Visit Checklist on page 34 (Figure 2-1) before each appointment, you will be well prepared.

In a typical office visit, your doctor is going to want to know certain pieces of information in a certain order: What has happened to you since the last office visit? What symptoms have you had? What symptoms are you currently having? How has the treatment worked? What side effects have you had? What laboratory tests have you had? How have you been faring emotionally? (Your Personal Health Log can be a great method of organizing this information between visits; see chapter 4.)

If you are prepared with even that much information, "we have a whole different consumer walking into that physician's office than we do if you think your job is to show up, shut up, and sit there," says Dr. Sherrie Kaplan. "We are really shifting some of the responsibility for preparation over to the patient, but to do any less, to shift it all to the doctor, is being very paternalistic."

And the more you know about your disease, the more you'll be able to prepare for the kinds of information the doctor will be looking for, including the symptoms that might be danger signs. For example, if you are suffering from a heart condition, your lower back pain will probably not be a very important clue about your health problem. But lower back pain can be a sign of metastasis to bone in a patient with advanced cancer, or a sign of kidney disease in a person with diabetes. The challenge is to understand enough to know what to look for without creating imaginary symptoms because you are so worried about them.

Because of time constraints, most doctors can handle only about three in-depth questions per visit, so put your questions in priority order. (Ask your doctor if you can fax or e-mail questions in advance of the visit. This will let your doctor know the scope of what you want to know, and may alert him or her to issues that haven't yet been brought up. This way, your doctor can prepare, too.) If you have many questions, try to answer some of them yourself with research, and save the more difficult questions for the expert. Remember, the examination and questions all have to be done in less than twenty minutes.

Interestingly, research has shown that doctors respond differently to active patients than to less-informed patients. "Physicians ask more questions and do more verifying when they are addressing the questions that trained patients ask," says Dr. Donald J. Cegala. That suggests that active patients require doctors to be more alert and on-the-ball than they might otherwise be. Sophisticated questions, after all, necessitate sophisticated answers.

Some important questions that patients often forget are:

- Is there another option for that treatment/test you've recommended?
- Which option offers the best chance of cure/pain relief/ remission?
- Which option holds the greatest risks?
- What are the likely short-term and long-term side effects?
- What have you seen in terms of success with that treatment?

▶ ACTION ITEM 7: *Bring additional information to a new doctor.*

If you are visiting a doctor for the first time, be sure to bring copies of your medical records, X-rays, CAT scans, or other test results. Much of the time in a first visit is spent reviewing records and determining exactly what the problem is. The more information you can provide, the more quickly you can move on to more profitable discussions about treatments. If you have a completed Personal Health Log (see chapter 4), bring it with you as well in case the physician wants to see details of your medical history.

▶ ACTION ITEM 8: *Participate in a support group or volunteer activities.*

Take advantage of any opportunity to learn more about your condition. "There is some evidence from studies that suggest that women [with breast cancer] who, for instance, are more active in support groups or active volunteering do better," says Dr. William C. Dooley of Johns Hopkins University Medical School. "It could be argued that that's because they are emotionally handling their disease better, but it could also be that they are seeking out better care, that they understand what the elements of good care are." The trick is to know which are valuable sources of information and which might be misleading or even damaging. (See chapter 14 for more information about support groups.)

▶ ACTION ITEM 9: *Be assertive when you need to be.*

There may be times when your newfound expertise in your own condition should allow you to take charge. "If a mother is taking care of a child with cystic fibrosis, and on the weekend she calls the general pediatrician on call, let's face it, she should pretty much be able to direct the care," says Dr. Sheldon Greenfield. But unless you have been to medical school, you can't ever assume that you know as much as a physician does. You know yourself, though. Once you understand your condition (or, in this example, the condition of your child), you've earned the right to help call the shots. Once you get to this point, ask your physician to write a note to put in your chart that explicitly states your ability to judge the need for certain care. That way, if your doctor is ever out of town and you need to continue treatments you are accustomed to dealing with, the doctor on-call will understand the situation.

The Doctor's Visit Checklist will help you organize your thoughts, prepare for the visit, and record information during a doctor's appointment. Complete as much of the form as you can prior to seeing your doctor, then refer back to it during the

visit. Photocopy and use this form to remind yourself of many
of the action items discussed in this chapter.

Figure 2-1. Doctor Visit Checklist
====

Doctor being seen:————————————————————
Date of visit:————————————————————
Reason for visit:————————————————————
Special concerns:————————————————————

If this is your first visit to a new doctor:
☐ Bring past medical records, including what treatments and
  tests you have had, the names of previous doctors, and, if
  possible, copies of your primary care physician's notes.
☐ Bring copies of X-rays, CAT scans, MRI films, blood test
  results, or other tests.
☐ Bring Personal Health Log (see chapter 4).

For any doctor visit:
☐ Bring list of all medications you are currently taking, including prescriptions, over-the-counter treatments (cold medicine,
  aspirin, or laxative), herbs, vitamins or other supplements.

Drug/supplement taken	*How often*	*Dosage*	*Any side effects*
————	————	————	————
————	————	————	————
————	————	————	————
————	————	————	————

☐ Bring written list of symptoms you have experienced since
  your last visit (add page, if necessary):

Symptom	*Type, severity, duration*	*Treatment, effectiveness*
————	————	————
————	————	————
————	————	————
————	————	————

☐ Write down the three most pressing questions you would like your doctor to answer:

1. _____
2. _____
3. _____

☐ Make sure you understand everything the doctor says, especially instructions. Ask the doctor to repeat or explain anything you didn't catch the first time.

☐ Write down instructions or information to look up for future reference.

Name of new medication prescribed:_____
   Instructions for taking:_____
   Side effects to watch for:_____
   How long until you'll see effects:_____

Name of new medication prescribed:_____
   Instructions for taking:_____
   Side effects to watch for:_____
   How long until you'll see effects:_____

Other special instructions:_____
   Anything you should be doing differently:_____
   Diet or behavior changes:_____
   Anything to prevent pain or side effects:_____

☐ If tests are recommended, ask if there are any risks to the tests and what you can do to minimize them. Ask what the doctor expects to learn from the test.

What are the tests:_____
When and where test is scheduled:_____
Special preparation needed:_____

☐ What is the best way to contact the doctor if you have further questions?_____

☐ Date of next appointment:_____

☐ If referred to another doctor, ask for copies of your medical records to be sent, or for your own copy to bring. Name of new doctor:_____

CONVERSATION STARTERS

Some patients are too shy or too afraid of offending their doctors to ask important questions. Others may feel that questioning will only make them look ignorant or foolish. In fact, the opposite is true. Use these "conversation starters" to ease your way into discussions you may otherwise feel uncomfortable about starting.

To open a discussion about partnering with your doctor:
[For any of these, if the doctor says no, find a new doctor!]
- "I want to become more active in my own health care. As part of this, I am searching for a doctor who will work with me in part-nership. Do you think we could have that type of relationship?"
- "Would you be comfortable with me taking a more active role in decision making?"
- "I am interested in shared medical decision making. Can we discuss how that would work in my case?"

To make sure you heard correctly or understood what was said:
- "Would you please repeat that?"
- "I don't know what you mean. Could you please explain that?"
- "Could you spell that?"
- "So, you think I should not worry about [some symptom or side effect]?"
- "OK, the name of the medicine was [repeat what you heard]. Is that correct?"
- "So, you are saying that I should [repeat instructions you heard]." Examples: "So, you are saying I should take three pills a day, one pill with each meal." Or, "I understood you to say that I should not do this exercise if it hurts when I do it."
- "I'm sorry, I still don't understand. Is there another way you could explain that?" Or, "Is there a nurse or physician's assistant who might be able to spend some time explaining that to me?"

To tell a doctor you are not happy with a treatment:
- "I know we discussed this treatment, but I'm having some diffi-culty following through. Here's why . . . [list your reasons]." For

example: "I'm having too many side effects," or, "I can't seem to take all those pills at the right time," or, "I really don't think it's helping me."
- "Is there another treatment option?"

To report something embarrassing:
- "This is hard for me to discuss, but you should know that [say it directly]."
- "I have a problem that is causing me some embarrassment."

To tell your doctor you'd like to get a second opinion:
- "I understand and respect what you are telling me, but for my own peace of mind, I would like to get a second opinion."
- "I feel comfortable with the options you have described, but as an informed consumer, I feel it is important to get a second opinion."
- "I may very well end up coming back here, but first I would like to get a second opinion."

To make sure your needs are met (choose the ones that are appropriate for you):
- To request taping an office visit: "I would like to tape record this conversation so that I can review the information later when I'm not so nervous. Would that be all right with you?"
- If your doctor starts to leave the office too soon: "I still have a couple of questions we haven't discussed . . . first, [ask your first question]." If the doctor does not have time for the questions, follow up with, "How can I get these questions answered? Is there a nurse who could help me?"
- If you have a journal article or other piece of information that you would like the doctor to comment on: "I found this piece of information about my condition. How might it apply to my situation?" or, "Would this be a treatment option we should consider?"
- If you want to try an alternative or complementary treatment: "I've heard about [name of alternative] as a treatment for my condition, and I was thinking about trying it. Do you see any reason why I should not try it?"

[Some questions reprinted with permission from "Communicating with Your Doctor," a patient-training booklet by Donald J. Cegala, Ph.D., of Ohio State University.]

3. You Need a System

LET'S say you were just diagnosed with diabetes and now want to learn everything you can about the disease. Ready . . . set . . . begin. . . .

According to the Library of Congress, there are 3,587 books on diabetes, and a certain proportion of these are written in a foreign language or deal with obscure aspects of the disease. Try Amazon.com instead, the consumer-friendly online bookstore. There you find a still-unreadable 1,433 entries for "diabetes." If you browse the Internet, you'll find more than 140 websites that deal in some way with diabetes, and an astounding 542,840 Web pages. The U.S. government's health directory, *healthfinder*™, which does an initial evaluation of websites, lists more than 50 Web resources and 24 diabetes organizations. Skip over to MEDLINE, the medical journal database, to peruse the latest information from medical journals (see chapter 9 for more information on MEDLINE). If you limit the scope of the search to studies of human beings, written in English, and printed since 1980, you'll still find more than 75,000 diabetes articles. And the numbers increase daily.

Clearly, you're going to need a strategy to know where to start, how to tell what's important to read and what isn't, and how to sort through the tens of thousands of pieces of information you're going to run into during your search. And after you have the specific information you need, you're going to want to have a convenient way to organize and store everything you've found. Without a strategy, it will be easy to get bogged down in the glut of health information out there, to be misled by rumors, to lose focus, or to repeat steps unnecessarily.

Forming an Information-Search Strategy

The strategy you use depends on the type of disease you have, how long you've had the disease, how much you already know, and how much time you can devote to your health search. Let's start by defining your illness. Which of the following three categories best describes your disorder?

ACUTE ILLNESS (MILD OR SEVERE)
Definition: Acute illnesses begin abruptly, have a relatively short course, then disappear either on their own or with medical help.

Examples: Allergic reaction, appendicitis, athlete's foot, blood clots, broken bones, bronchitis, ear infections, food poisoning, heart attack, influenza, poison ivy rash, strep throat, stroke, vaginal yeast infections. These problems happen, and go away with time, rest, antibiotics, surgery, or other treatment.

Information-gathering strategy: None—it won't help in these situations. You can always search for information, but you don't need much in the way of a strategy. You may not have time to do the research, and often the treatments are so standard that there is very little to challenge. Exception: If your doctor warns you that you are at high risk for heart attack, stroke, or some other acute problem, follow the "Methodical Strategy" below to learn how to prevent these serious outcomes.

Continuity: If these conditions recur (allergic reactions, infections, or athlete's foot), they can be treated as manageable chronic conditions, with information gathering focused on searching for a way to prevent the condition in the future (use "Methodical Strategy"). Heart attack and stroke are, in themselves, acute problems. But the residual disease or disability should be treated as a life-threatening chronic condition. Information gathering in those cases should focus on preventing future attacks and dealing with the effects of the original attack (use "Urgent Strategy").

CHRONIC ILLNESS (LIFE-THREATENING)

Definition: A chronic illness develops slowly and persists for a long time, sometimes throughout the rest of a person's life. Life-threatening chronic illnesses can take months or years to develop, but once discovered and diagnosed, they require relatively quick and decisive action to prevent death.

Examples: Any type of cancer, heart disease, brain tumors, HIV/AIDS.

Information-gathering strategy: "Urgent Strategy."

Continuity: Once initial treatment has begun, a life-threatening illness may become a manageable illness. When the time of crisis that requires quick action has passed, switch to "Methodical Strategy" to learn disease management and to maintain awareness of the latest treatments should there be a relapse.

CHRONIC ILLNESS (MANAGEABLE)

Definition: These are diseases that develop slowly and persist for a long time but are not immediately life-threatening. They can be mild or very serious. Some have cyclic periods of flare-ups and remissions, some require a constant level of care, and others are increasingly debilitating over time.

Examples: Allergies, Alzheimer's disease, amyotrophic lateral sclerosis (ALS), asthma, cirrhosis, Crohn's disease, diabetes, epilepsy, gastroesophageal reflux disease (heartburn), hepatitis C, hypoglycemia, Lyme disease, mental illnesses, migraines, multiple sclerosis, muscular dystrophy, neurofibromatosis, osteoarthritis, Parkinson's disease, psoriasis, rheumatoid arthritis, thyroid problems, systemic lupus erythematosus, ulcerative colitis.

Information-gathering strategy: Patients newly diagnosed with a chronic manageable disease may want to start with the "Urgent Strategy" to gain a quick understanding of what is happening and what treatment options are available. Once the disease is under control, or if the patient has already had the disease for a while, the "Methodical Strategy" will allow a broader and deeper understanding of the disease.

Continuity: Managing a chronic disease may require changing treatment strategies several times over the years. Patients who do not keep track of the latest information about their diseases may miss out on state-of-the-art treatments, especially if they have paternalistic or entrenched physicians. Informed active patients will be the first to benefit when new medications are approved or new ways to manage the disease are developed. The solution: Do periodic searches on the Internet for organizational information, and check the medical journal database MEDLINE for the latest information. (See chapter 9 for more information on MEDLINE searches.) Depending on your disease and how much time you'd like to devote to keeping abreast of research, these can be done weekly, monthly, or yearly. Common diseases get more funding and are more likely to have regular major announcements and research reports. For example, in a single month, a search of medical journals revealed that 457 articles were published about heart disease, 187 for breast cancer, and 76 for prostate cancer, but only 12 for neurofibromatosis and 9 for meningiomas. Recheck for common disease information weekly or monthly. For less common diseases, you can limit your search to once every six months to a year.

The Methodical Strategy

The Methodical Strategy for health information gathering allows you to become an expert in your disease by absorbing available information in a systematic and measured way. This can be done in as little as two months of full-time work (if you have the flexibility to take that much time off from work), or it can be a lifetime project. Use it if:

- You want to have a firm knowledge of your condition, *and*
- You don't have an immediate treatment decision to make, *and*
- You need to manage your disease over a long period of time, or
- You want to prevent a recurrence of mild acute illnesses, such as infections.

The main benefit of the Methodical Strategy is that you will know nearly as much as—in some cases, more than—your doctor about your condition. Your knowledge will be well-grounded and you will be highly prepared to share medical decision making. The main drawback is that it will take a considerable amount of time. (But remember, this kind of investment will most likely pay off later in the form of better health, better quality of life, and more control over your treatment. See Figure 3-1).

As you can see in the diagram, the Methodical Strategy for information gathering follows a linear route, starting from the most basic information found in books. You don't need to read everything available. Start by reading one or two books all the way through; once you feel you've absorbed the basic information, then move on to the next stage. As you work your way through progressively more detailed information, you reach the most complex form of health information (the medical journal). Think of it as going through grammar school and middle school before heading off to high school . . . by the time you get there, you'll be well prepared.

Once you understand your condition well enough, talk to other people who have had the same disease and doctors or researchers who specialize in the exact type of problem you have. By the time you've read through all the material available, you'll know who the experts in your disease are, you'll be

Figure 3-1. Methodical Strategy

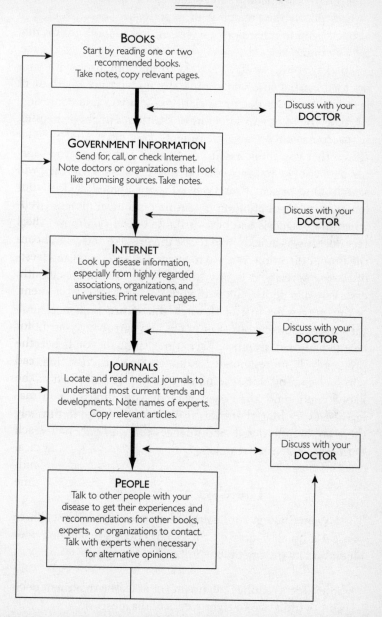

able to discern good information from bad, and you'll be able to listen to other people's treatment stories and know how well or how poorly they match your experience. These people can also lead you to other books, websites, and support groups that they've found helpful.

The key to this strategy is to keep touching back with your doctor to make sure you completely understand what you're learning. Ask your doctor to clarify points you find confusing, to guide you to other sources he or she thinks might be helpful, or to comment on new treatments you discovered in your search that you think might be appropriate for you. Your doctor can also help keep you on the right track during your search. One patient I interviewed spent a good deal of time looking up information on inflammatory bowel disease (IBD) when her diagnosis had been irritable bowel syndrome (IBS). Her doctor was quickly able to see the mistake and point her in the proper direction. With so many grades and stages and levels of disease severity, it is easy to lose focus of your specific disease. When in doubt, talk with your doctor.

You may want to run through this entire sequence more than once, choosing different books and narrowing your Internet and journal searches. Each time through you'll become progressively more knowledgeable about your condition, and will feel comfortable reading more complex information. It's likely you'll find that even though you thought you had learned everything there was to know the first time through, there are helpful details and nuances that can only be learned with more extensive searches.

The Urgent Strategy

The Urgent Strategy for health information gathering will help you get a quick handle on the major issues surrounding your illness and its treatment. Use it if:

- Your illness requires treatment (or at least a treatment decision) within two to eight weeks of diagnosis, or

- You've been diagnosed with a serious illness and immediately want to know as much as possible in order to start treatment or get a handle on what you're dealing with, or
- You need to prevent a recurrence of a serious acute illness (such as heart attack or stroke), or
- You have otherwise very limited time and are willing to sacrifice depth of knowledge for basic understanding.

The main benefit of the Urgent Strategy is that you are able to get a lot of information in a very short amount of time. Think of it as a massive data-dump into your brain. The main drawback is that it requires nonlinear thinking. While the Methodical Strategy follows an easy progression from Point A to Point B to Point C, the Urgent Strategy requires you to jump around from point to point, sometimes doing several searches simultaneously. Imagine needing to bake a loaf of bread, a batch of cookies, and a cake all at the same time. You'd have to keep track of three different recipes, use several different mixing bowls, measure out common ingredients at the same time, and have them ready to bake simultaneously in the oven. Needless to say, unless you are very organized, things can become quite chaotic and the paperwork can get out of control. But if you need the information fast, this is the best way to go. (If you are uncomfortable with this type of multiple projects work, try doing a Methodical Strategy but skim the books for valuable keywords to search with, and skip ahead to the next phase as soon as you feel you're ready.)

As you can see in Figure 3-2, the Urgent Strategy begins with contacting people, basically sending out a network-wide S-O-S to gather help wherever you can. While the Methodical Strategy suggests having conversations with other people as the culmination point, the Urgent Strategy saves time by relying on the experience of others. The first step is to tell everyone you know about your diagnosis. Ask if they know anyone who has had the same disease, or if they have heard of a good doctor who specializes in your disease. Unless you have an extremely rare illness, chances are you'll collect several names very quickly.

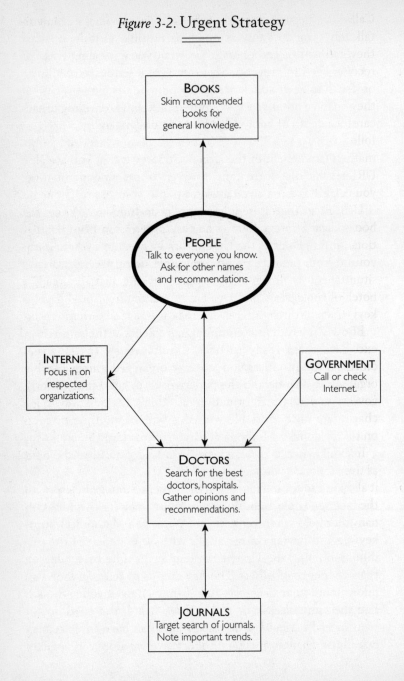

Figure 3-2. Urgent Strategy

BOOKS
Skim recommended
books for
general knowledge.

PEOPLE
Talk to everyone you know.
Ask for other names
and recommendations.

INTERNET
Focus in on
respected
organizations.

GOVERNMENT
Call or check
Internet.

DOCTORS
Search for the best
doctors, hospitals.
Gather opinions and
recommendations.

JOURNALS
Target search of journals.
Note important trends.

Call these individuals and ask them if they would be willing to talk with you about their experiences, their treatment, what they've learned, and what sources of information they would recommend. Specifically, ask if there were any books, websites, or organizations that they found particularly helpful, and if they worked with any doctors they would recommend. Keep careful notes during these conversations in case you need to follow up. And don't be afraid to ask for as much specific information as you can get—phone numbers, addresses, website URLs, photocopies of journal articles. Save time wherever you can.

Use those recommendations (and the information in this book) to choose one or two books to skim for relevant information. Your goals are to get an overview of the major issues of your disease, and to find specific keywords that apply to your situation or to potential treatments. Write them down in a notebook. When you have five or more focused questions or keywords, move on to the Internet.

Books are great for in-depth information, but the Internet excels at providing "sound bites" of information. Use sites recommended by the people you spoke with, or locate reputable organizations that specialize in your disease (see chapter 10), government institutes (see chapter 7), and journal articles (see chapter 9). Read some of the general information, then search on the specific keywords that apply to your condition.

In the beginning, print or copy everything you see that looks as though it pertains to your situation. You may not understand it all initially, but it will make more sense as you begin to put all the information together. The more you read, the more certain names or issues will pop out at you. Use these as additional keywords to guide further searches. (See chapter 8 for more information on searching the Internet.) Touch back to each type of information source as often as you need to. Place all information in the appropriate spot in your Personal Health Log (see chapter 4), and refer back to it often.

After you have absorbed the major issues, look for physician experts. When you spoke with other patients and your primary care physician, did any names pop up more than once? Who wrote the books you read? Who seemed to be mentioned in journal articles most often? These are probably the "big guns" in your area. If possible, make an appointment to talk with one or two of these specialists about your case. If you don't already have a local specialist you would like to use, think of these meetings as job interviews to see who you might like to work with to help manage your health. Before you meet with them, make sure you have a good understanding of your condition and that you've outlined the pros and cons of various treatments for yourself. In other words, be especially prepared before your meeting if you want to get the most benefit from the limited amount of time you'll have with these experts. If you can't get an appointment with one of the big guns, ask for the name of a doctor they respect.

The key to this search is to realize that you are looking for nuggets of information that can provide you with enough understanding to make the best medical decisions you can make in the face of stress and illness. When you're racing against the clock to treat a brain tumor, for example, you don't necessarily need to know how the tumor got there, or all the different types of brain tumors there are, or the history of brain tumor diagnosis. You need to know—for your specific brain tumor—what the treatment options are, what the real risks and benefits of each are, what follow-up or experimental treatments might be available, and which doctors and hospitals are the best at treating your type of tumor.

URGENT STRATEGY: ARTHUR, PROSTATE CANCER

When Arthur was diagnosed with a relatively early stage prostate cancer at the end of May 1999, he gave himself two months to research all his treatment options, talk with specialists, and decide which treatment would be best for him. His search is a textbook example of an Urgent Search. He tells it in his own words:

The diagnosis of prostate cancer basically gave me a new identity, a new way to start thinking about my life. I was now a man with stage T2b prostate cancer, Gleason grade 6, with a PSA of 3.1 [prostate specific antigen, a blood test, which, if it reaches a level over 4.0, is suspicious for prostate cancer]. Just that little bit of information was enough for me to start my information search.

It's important to understand that with hindsight things seem more rational, planned, orderly, and thoughtful than they really were. In reality, you pursue a lot of things simultaneously, there's a lot of chaos, a lot of things going on at once—phone calls, meetings, reading. It would be very easy to say, after the fact, "Oh, gee, he had a real process." I'm not sure that I really did. I just did what seemed right.

First thing I did was get some big notebooks and start writing down lists of people I knew. Did I know anybody who had prostate cancer? It turned out that I did, a friend of the family, younger than me, who had gone through this several years earlier. I called him up and found that, like almost anybody who has gone through this, he was extremely willing to talk and help. He gave me the name of his medical oncologist, who had written a book about prostate cancer. So of course I started checking up on this guy and his credentials. I immediately got his book out of our local public library and thought it was good. I called a couple of other people, some doctors, and they all said that, yes, they had heard of him, and that he had a good reputation. So right away, within three to four days, I had one potential person I might use as a medical oncologist.

I also told a huge number of friends and relatives what I was going through, and asked if they knew anybody who had the disease who might be willing to talk to me. In the month of June, I got to talk at length (sometimes for up to ninety minutes) with six people, all perfect strangers, who had been treated for prostate cancer within the last six or seven years.

At the same time, I continued looking for potential doctors to work with. I knew my main choices of treatment were surgery or radiation, so I wanted to find good surgeons and radiation oncologists who specialized in prostate cancer, as well as a medical oncologist to oversee my case. I called almost every physician my wife and I knew. In the first couple of weeks, I called about ten different doctors, just asking for recommendations of those types of physicians, or other doctors I might call who could make a recommendation. I spent a lot of time on the phone.

At this point, I found myself very much in the middle of a gradual information overload. I was learning from reading (I read five or six books), I surfed the Net, and I talked with all these people. My immediate concern wasn't just in finding the "best surgeon" or the best "radiation person." I had to figure out whether surgery or radiation was the better treatment. That's a much bigger question, and it took a lot of reading.

In deciding treatment for this disease, there are a couple of considerations. First, of course, is which procedure might best cure you. But the flip side is that there are tremendous long-range side effects from any procedure. [Impotence and incontinence are two common side effects of treatment for prostate cancer.] So you also have to ask, given who you are, with your values, which procedure not only is most likely to cure you, but which will produce the least damaging long-term side effects from your point of view.

I spent a lot of time looking at what books were available, going to Amazon.com, asking people for their recommendations. After a while, I discovered I could quickly recognize which Internet sites were primarily commercial, promoting something like herbal remedies or selling a hospital, and which gave unbiased information.

I also discovered that it was possible to get into the recent issues of some leading medical journals and look at articles, usually just the summaries but sometimes the whole article. I knew that if one of the summaries looked interesting, my local hospital had a library that was available to somebody like me. I could walk in, find an article, copy it, and try to make sense out of it.

By the end of June, I realized that I didn't have the rest of my life to make a decision. I had to begin making appointments to see some specialists, especially since you can't just pick up the phone and get an appointment the next day with most of these physicians.

Before my appointments, I summarized all the information about my condition on one page: who I am, my condition, age, stage, and so on, followed by my questions. Doctors love that because it makes their job a little easier. And it meant they could tailor their comments to their sense of how ignorant or how up-to-speed I was about my condition. Several of the doctors said that after reading my summary, they could assume that I knew certain things, and that they didn't have to tell me over and over and over again the same thing they would say to somebody walking in cold, ignorant of the disease.

None of the doctors would tell me what to do—it was too close a call. There wasn't a definitive answer. I had a few more consultations with different types of specialists, I did more research, and by the end of July, it was time to make a decision. I still was not 100 percent sure what to do, but for a number of reasons I chose surgery.

Before settling on a surgeon, however, I had to do more research. I checked credentials, where they went to medical school, and how many surgeries of this type they had done. There's tremendous variation among skill levels of physicians, and one of the hardest things to figure out if you are a patient is who is really good and who isn't. I found someone I was comfortable with, who gave me confidence in his surgical skills, and had the surgery on September 16, 1999.

I still don't know if I really made the right choice from the point of view of getting rid of the disease. So far, so good. The pathology after the operation was good. And my PSA is down to 0.

For me, this was an enormously big, profound deal. We're talking about life and death and all that. I realized that it was up to me . . . I had to take the bull by the horns. You have to do your own due diligence, knowing that you're always dealing with limited knowledge.

I didn't read all the books, I didn't see all the oncologists I wanted to. Still, I gathered a lot of information, filling four college notebooks, and I have a stack of copied journal articles about two and a half feet high on a shelf in my bedroom. I learned enough to make an informed decision, even though there isn't necessarily a single "right" answer from a medical perspective. The decision also depends on personal preferences, how you feel about various side effects—no doctor can tell you that. So you have to learn a little bit about yourself as a by-product of learning about your disease.

4. Your Personal Health Log

IF we all had photographic memories, we could read a book once and later recall every word. It wouldn't be necessary to take notes, make copies, or organize the information. Sadly, few of us have that ability. In fact, if you talk to anyone over age thirty-five, chances are they'll say their memories seem more like sieves than catch-basins.

Some doctors estimate that patients recall only about 20 percent of everything they hear in a doctor's office. The physical and emotional strain of dealing with an illness wreaks havoc with our memories—we forget more easily, or sometimes add additional information that isn't really there, "reading between the lines" to suit our own sense of optimism or pessimism. Would you bet your life on a set of half-remembered facts? Would you want to choose a medical treatment if you couldn't remember what the side effects might be? The best decisions are made when you have all the facts laid out in front of you, easily accessible. In short, once you find the information, you need a way to organize it.

The Personal Health Log is one way to get and stay organized. It will be an ongoing record of your medical condition, the disease information you find, and your treatment history. You can bring it to your doctor to show your progress, or to a new doctor to bring him or her up to speed on your condition. It will take some time to put together initially, but once you have the basic format laid out, the Personal Health Log will save you time by organizing all your health information in one place.

Step-by-step guidelines for creating a Personal Health Log (PHL) are listed below. Blank forms (templates) for each section are provided later in this chapter, on pages 61 to 67. Simply photocopy as many pages as you need, and start filling them out.

As you gain experience in keeping the log, you may find that you need to add new sections for information specific to your disease, or that you can remove sections that don't apply to you. Feel free to customize the log in a way that allows you the best access to information.

So, let's get organized.

What You'll Need

- Three-ring binder (at least one inch deep, with interior pockets)
- Paper
- Tab pages (eight tabs needed)
- Access to a photocopier and three-hole paper-punch, usually available at a local library or office supply superstore, such as Staples or OfficeMax
- Spiral notebook, any size you find convenient to keep with you

Keep a notebook with you at all times to mark down information wherever you are—at your desk, on a bus, or at the library. Don't carry your PHL with you except to the doctor's office. If it gets lost, you'll lose a lot of time and valuable information. Transfer important information from the notebook to your PHL.

Personal Health Log Guidelines

For any section, if all your information won't fit on the form provided, make additional copies or write the extra information on a separate piece of paper that you keep with the form. Copy completed forms as needed to give to your physician. If you find an exciting article or other piece of information but don't have the time to file it in your PHL, put the information in the pocket inside the front cover of the binder to make sure it stays safe until you can get around to placing it where it belongs.

SECTIONS TO COMPLETE IMMEDIATELY

"Physician Information" form: This form will be the first page in your binder, acting as your handy contact page and as a reference you can give to your physicians in case they need to contact each other.

"Condition Summary" form: The second form in your PHL asks you to list specific disease information, as well as all medications, surgeries, or treatments that have been completed or tried to date. This form serves two main purposes: *First*, it will contain the basic information you need in order to begin a health information search. If you cannot complete this form on your own, bring it to your doctor and ask for help. Be as specific as possible. For example, if you received chemotherapy, find out the exact name of the chemotherapy drug you used and the dosage given. (See "Do I Know This?," page 60.)

Second, it will be a convenient way to communicate your condition history with any new doctor you consult. On these two pages (or one page if you make two-sided copies), your doctor will have all the basic information about your condition, saving you a lot of time during the office visit. Update this form at least once each year.

SECTIONS TO COMPLETE THROUGHOUT THE YEAR

After the Physician Information and Condition Summary forms, make your first tab. Although the tabs may seem unnecessary in the beginning, once your PHL grows, you'll need to have important sections clearly marked so you can turn to them quickly.

Make a tab marked "Appointments"

"Appointment Chart" form: This form will be an ongoing history of your medical care from now on. Mark every appointment on the chart and fill in the boxes according to the headers. Use the last box for any reminders, results, or personal comments about the test, procedure, or visit. This information may also come in handy for completing insurance forms.

"Doctor Visit Checklist" (see Chapter 2, Figure 2-1): Keep completed checklists to refer back to later. Keep a supply of blank checklists for future visits.

Make a tab marked "Symptoms"

"Symptom Chart" form: This form will be an ongoing history of your symptoms. For every symptom you feel, make an entry according to the headers. When describing the symptom, be as specific as possible. For example, if you have pain, describe exactly where the pain is located and what the pain feels like (see "Symptom Descriptors," page 60). Include emotional symptoms as well as physical ones. If the symptom appears several times in one day, you don't need to make separate notations—just indicate the different times in the "Duration" box. If you do anything to try to stop the symptoms, no matter how silly you might think it is, write it down (especially if it helps). What works or doesn't work may serve as an important clue for your doctor.

Make a tab marked "Treatments"

"Treatment Information" form: Use this form to chart medications, physical therapy, radiation, massage, or other treatments you receive.

• For medications, include both brand and generic names of the drug. Under "Date," write the date you start taking the drug. Write the dosage, how often to take the drug, and how long to take it in the third column. Complete all other boxes if applicable.

• For other treatments, complete as many boxes as you can. If you are prescribed a series of identical treatments, as might be the case with radiation or physical therapy sessions, you don't need to complete the chart each time you have a treatment, just note the different dates in the "Date" box or write a note about the treatment series in the "Dosage" box.

Make a tab marked "Monitoring"

"Monitoring Chart" form: Adapt and use this chart to keep track of certain medical readings or behaviors, such as blood pressure or blood glucose readings, diet, exercise or smoking habits. Have a separate chart for each thing you want to monitor. Write what you will be monitoring in the blank at the top of the page, then complete a new row each time you take a reading. (If you need to measure more than once a day, as you would for blood glucose, write the date and time in the "Date" box.) Put the actual reading in the box marked "Status," such as blood pressure, weight, number of cigarettes smoked, and any description and problems or extenuating circumstances in the "Comments" box. If you don't have to watch for anything, then this section can be eliminated.

Make a tab marked "My Journal"

Put twenty blank pages in this section to start, then add more pages as you begin to fill them up. Use this section to "talk through" your thoughts on the pros and cons of various treatment options that you discover during your information search. If you read two books and ten journal articles, it can be very difficult to remember all the different options presented. Although most patients are not used to thinking of their feelings as important to their disease process, your personal feelings, beliefs, and values will play an important role in the treatment decision-making process. It is also a good place to note favorite information sources to which you might want to return later. Specific information to note:

- Treatments you read about that seem particularly optimistic or pessimistic. What makes them noteworthy to you?
- Percentages or other statistics that you want to remember. For example, if 100 percent of patients who survive a particular procedure are cured, but 50 percent of patients don't survive the procedure, those are significant numbers that can lead different people to different conclusions and decisions. Mark where you read the information so you can refer back to it later. How did you feel about it when you first read the information? Did your thoughts change over time?
- Lists of pros and cons of various treatment options, from your perspective.
- Websites you would like to remember, especially if they post new information regularly.
- Lists of books read: titles, authors, publishers, and dates of publication, along with any thoughts you had about the value of each book. A year from now you may want to reread a particular book, and this way you'll have the exact title of the one you found so helpful.

SECTIONS FOR DOCUMENTS

Make a tab marked "Physician Reports"

Every time your physician receives a report from a biopsy, blood test, X-ray, or other procedure, he or she receives a written report of the results. Ask for copies of each report and file them in this section. Although your doctor should give you a verbal summary of what is in the report and what it means for you, it is always valuable to have your own copy to refer back to, or to bring to a new doctor in case you need an additional consultation or if your doctor is away but you need immediate attention during an emergency.

Read through the reports before your next visit, and ask your doctor to clarify any information you don't understand. Some of the information will be presented in a way that looks confusing, but it's actually rather easy to understand once the laboratory "shorthand" has been explained. For example, blood test results are reported as a single number for each test, with a range of numbers that are considered "normal." If your number falls within the range, no matter what the test, you really don't have to worry about it. Ask your doctor about any test results that fall outside the "normal" range, and what those readings might mean for you.

Other information, such as X-ray or MRI reports, are presented as a written report from one doctor to another. These are often filled with medical jargon and can be difficult to understand. Read through them with a medical dictionary at your side, and write normal-language definitions in pencil above any confusing words or phrases. Read it through again, and ask your doctor about any information that still seems confusing or seems to conflict with what he or she told you during the summary.

Make a tab marked "Journal Articles"

This is the place to store copies of articles you find particularly helpful or insightful. Keep less relevant articles in a separate location or throw them away. You don't need to clutter up your PHL with unimportant information. If you have a very common disorder that has generated a lot of research, you may need to find a more extensive filing system. Some systems that work for other people include: bigger binders with tabs to separate articles into subcategories, file folders stored in drawers or file boxes, and stacks of articles on bookshelves or in boxes.

Make a tab marked "To Save or File"

Consider this your catchall tab. As you go about your search, you'll run across a lot of information you'll want to save for future reference, such as brochures, letters from friends or other patients, Web pages you've printed out, newspaper clippings, and other items. Put everything you think is important in this section by punching holes in it (as for brochures and Web pages), or by taping or pasting the item onto blank paper (as for newspaper articles). This section will fill up fast, so clear it out regularly—as you learn more and more about your illness, you'll find that what you thought was once important enough to save is now outdated or seems like simple common knowledge.

CHECKLIST: DO I KNOW THIS?

When creating your PHL, here are some guidelines to follow to ensure that the information you include will be clear and complete. If there are any questions you cannot answer, check with your doctor. The answers are important to your information search and your general understanding of your condition:

☐ What is the full name of my disease or condition?
☐ What stage, grade, or severity is it? (if appropriate)
☐ What medications am I currently taking?
    ☐ What are their names? (get brand *and* generic name)
    ☐ What are they supposed to do?
    ☐ What side effects are common?
☐ What other treatment options are available aside from the one(s) I am doing?
☐ What are the pros and cons, risks and benefits of all my options?
☐ How would my doctor like to be contacted if I have a question?
☐ Is there a nurse or physician's assistant generally available for questions?

SYMPTOM DESCRIPTORS

Pain can be:
Sharp, dull, pounding, jabbing, grabbing, hot, burning, achy, throbbing, deep, heavy, localized to one spot, all-over
Body part can feel:
Numb, tingly, "buzzing," hot, cold, swollen, bloated, weak, shaky, trembling, crampy, tender, tight, weak
Stomach can be:
Queasy, nauseated, vomiting, cramping, bloated
Symptom can be:
Constant, intermittent, persistent, occasional, rare

Figure 4-1. Personal Health Log of _____
(Name)

Physician Information
Primary care physician: _____
    Phone number: _____
    Fax: _____
    Address: _____

    E-mail address: _____
Specialist: _____
    Area of specialty: _____
    Phone number: _____
    Fax: _____
    Address: _____

    E-mail address: _____
Specialist: _____
    Area of specialty: _____
    Phone number: _____
    Fax: _____
    Address: _____

    E-mail address: _____
Specialist: _____
    Area of specialty: _____
    Phone number: _____
    Fax: _____
    Address: _____

    E-mail address: _____

Figure 4-2. Condition Summary

Name of condition:_____
  Specific type:_____
  Status/Severity:_____
  Other categories:_____
  Complications?:_____
Date diagnosed:_____
Age at diagnosis:_____
Physician who diagnosed:_____
Diagnostic tests performed:_____
_____

List other chronic conditions:_____

List **all** medications, vitamins, herbs, over-the-counter drugs,
or other products you currently take:

Name of product	*Dosage*	*How often?*	*Any side effects?*

List any medications you tried for this condition **in the past**
(include chemotherapy):

Name of product	*Dosage*	*How often?*	*Any side effects?*

List medication allergies:_____

List all surgeries and hospital stays:

Surgery	*Reason*	*Date/Hospital*
_____	_____	_____
_____	_____	_____
_____	_____	_____
_____	_____	_____
_____	_____	_____

List any other treatments completed or tried (include physical therapy, radiation, acupuncture, massage, immobilization, or anything else not already listed above. Give as many details as possible, including when you had it, duration of treatment, how well it worked, side effects, etc.).

_____

_____

_____

_____

_____

Do you currently smoke? ____Yes ____No
Did you smoke in the past? ____Yes ____No
When did you quit smoking?:_____
Have you made any changes to your diet or exercise routine as a result of your condition? ____Yes ____No
If yes, describe how:

_____

_____

_____

_____

_____

Figure 4-3. Appointment Chart

Physician or procedure	Date	Location	Comments

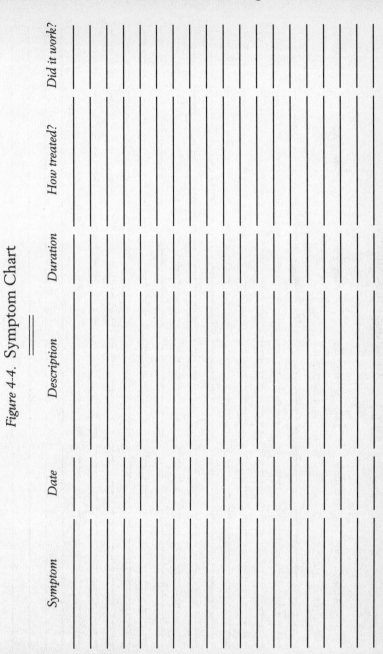

Figure 4-4. Symptom Chart

Symptom	Date	Description	Duration	How treated?	Did it work?

Figure 4-5. Treatment Information

Medication or Treatment	Date	Dosage/Amount and duration	Purpose	Side effects	Outcome

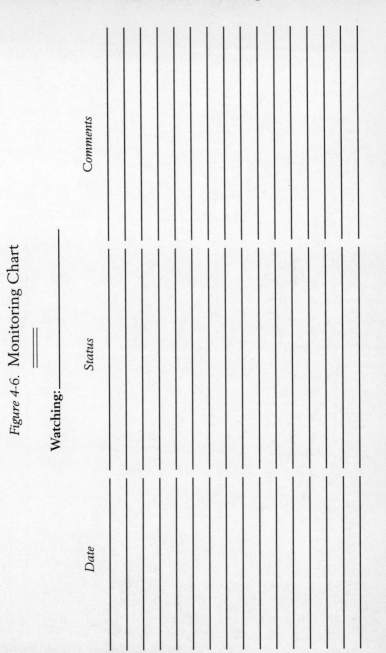

Figure 4-6. Monitoring Chart

Watching: _____

| Date | Status | Comments |

Information Sources

5. Books

Value as a health information source: ★ ★ ★ ☆
Effort required: ★ ★ ☆ ☆
Accessibility: ★ ★ ★ ★

Assessment: A good starting point for general information. The best source of in-depth information, although not necessarily state of the art.

FOR all but the rarest of illnesses, books can be a patient's most valuable source of information and comfort. Although they require more of a time commitment than other resources, books give you "breathing room." They provide the space to explore the background, intricacies, and nuances of a disease. Books can tell the complete story with examples and testimonials, photographs and illustrations, references and footnotes. They are the written equivalent of a full-length movie, while a magazine article is commercial-length and the Internet is made up of sound bites of information.

Many patients speak with passion about how books helped them learn, understand, and cope with their illnesses. After choosing carefully, and reading several, most patients tend to settle on one or two that they feel are the most useful. Once they select their favorites, they tend not to let those books out of their sight.

What keeps books from getting a "four-star" rating for value as an information source is the time-lag problem. Books take a long time to write—six months to a year, and sometimes longer, depending on the book and the writer. And they take at least that amount of time to be edited and printed. The rule of thumb is that it takes as long to publish a book as it does to carry a baby to term—about nine months from the time the writer finishes the manuscript until it is available in bookstores and libraries. This means that by the time you see a book, the words were written at least one to two years earlier.

For information that doesn't change in the short-run, this publishing time lag does not affect the quality of the book. For example, information about different types of cancer, or how to prevent an asthma attack, or how nutrition might help heart disease will remain valuable for many years. After all, basic anatomy and disease mechanisms don't change from year to year. Books can also reliably give solid information about most common treatment options, especially those that are proved to be successful in scientific research. These types of treatments will likely remain viable options for many years. And books that provide comforting stories, examples of treatment successes and cures, never go out of date.

But for information that is likely to change quickly, the publishing time lag has considerable consequences. For this reason, no book can claim to contain a comprehensive list of disease treatments or resources because new treatments, books, and websites are constantly being developed. By the time the book is published, some items are already bound to be missing that weren't even created or discovered when the book was written. This is unavoidable. For example, one cancer patient discovered a book that listed the various potential side effects associated with specific chemotherapy treatments. His first chemotherapy drug was included, and the suggestions for dealing with the side effects were tremendously helpful, but the chemotherapy drug used in the next round of treatments was too new to have been included in the book. Within six months, the book lost its value for that patient. And because of the rapid changes that occur in the Internet, some websites listed in a book may have disappeared by the time you try to find them. This does not mean that the book was "bad," that the author was uninformed, or that all of the information should be discounted, just that the fast-changing information became outdated. For more recent information, you'll need to search the Internet (see chapter 8) or read medical journals (see chapter 9).

Types of Health Books

All health books are not equal. Not only are there different categories of books, but like all information sources, some are more complete, more accurate, or more reliable than others.

Many patients find that they want and need different types of books at different points during their treatment. For example, newly diagnosed patients may want to read a disease-specific book first to understand what is happening to them, then start an inspirational book to help overcome the emotional aspects of the disease. Even later, they may want to find a medical textbook to understand their disease more fully.

GENERAL MEDICAL GUIDES

These books are the equivalent of a user's manual for the human body and are excellent resources for anyone, sick or not. Although each guide will vary slightly in its content, simplicity, and detail, medical guides generally contain information about disease prevention, nutrition, exercise, diagnostic tests, specific diseases, how the body works, first aid, and when to see the doctor.

If you have been diagnosed with an illness, this type of book will be of limited value for information about your particular disease, since most entries tend to be short. But medical guides can provide a simple snapshot look at your disorder that may be helpful to someone who is newly diagnosed or is just beginning an information search. In other words, it's a place to start to become generally familiar with the basics of an illness. If you take the time to read through some of the other sections of the book, however, you'll find an abundance of solid information

about other health issues that may help in your battle against
your illness. For example, good nutrition, adding exercise to
your life, and other typically "preventive" measures can be used
by just about anyone to improve overall health.

Go to a large bookstore, such as Barnes & Noble or Borders,
and browse through their selection of general medical guides.
You can always order books through your favorite outlet or
shop, but you really need hands-on experience with these
books in order to choose the one that's best for you. Once
there . . .

• *Pick the book up.* They vary in size from about 7 x 9.5 inches
to 9 x 11 inches—and the larger the book, the heavier it is. If
you are going to keep the book out on a reading table, weight
will make no difference. But some of these guides are so large
and heavy that it can be difficult to take them down off a shelf,
and if a book is too cumbersome, you won't use it. Choose one
you can physically handle with ease.

• *Look for one that has been published within the last four years.*
Any older than that and the information won't be current
enough to be useful. New guides and new editions of old
guides are constantly being published, so there will always be
several to choose from.

• *Check what additional supporting material is provided with
the guide.* Some now come with a free CD-ROM or provide
Internet updates. If these are important to you, factor them
into your decision.

• *Flip through the book and look at the style.* Some books provide full-color photographs of disease examples, others provide
detailed line drawings. See which appeals to you most. Some
people don't want to see all the gory details of diseases they'll
never have every time they open a book, while others love to
see rashes and other body dysfunctions in realistic color.

• *Examine the entries for the same disease in several books.* See
which book provides the kind of information you need most.
Some books tend to focus on the background of the disease,
why it happened, while others focus on what symptoms might

be useful for diagnosis, while still others spend more time talking about treatment. Choose the book that provides the level of detail you need.

• *Check the organization that participated in putting the book together.* Most medical guides are written by, or in cooperation with, large medical institutions or associations. If you run across one that isn't, pass it by. For example, the best medical guides on the shelves today (as of this writing) are the *American Medical Association Family Medical Guide*, the *American College of Physicians Complete Home Medical Guide*, the *Johns Hopkins Family Health Book*, the *Harvard Medical School Family Health Guide*, and the *Merck Manual of Medical Information—Home Edition*. No doubt other organizations will write equally good guides in future years.

CONSUMER-ORIENTED DISEASE-SPECIFIC BOOKS

These "specialty" books narrow the range of focus to a single disease or category of disease. Because these books are written specifically for patients, the language is usually easily understood and the explanations are detailed and clear. For this reason, they are a terrific source of in-depth information. Although each book will cover the material differently, specialty books often provide background information about the disease, anatomical and physiological explanations, diagnostic procedures, treatment options, self-help options, psychological and emotional guidance, quality-of-life guidance, and resources.

If you have a common disorder, you'll have a great many books from which to choose. Cancer, heart disease, diabetes, multiple sclerosis, arthritis, AIDS, endometriosis, asthma, allergies, Alzheimer's disease, headaches, and eating disorders are among the most popular book topics. Rare disorders will have fewer or sometimes no specialty books devoted to them. There may be a book that deals with a multitude of rare diseases, or a chapter about a rare disease in a category-wide specialty book, but you'll have to search the book index or table of contents to know if your disease is covered. For example, there is no consumer-oriented book that deals specifically with ischemic colitis, but information about that disease may be found in a more general book on gastrointestinal diseases.

Look for:

• *Books that are not more than four years old*. These are more likely to have relatively current information.

• *Classics*. These are the books that have gone into second or third (or more) editions. Your best bet is a book that is in an advanced edition, and that has been "revised" or "expanded" (it will say so on the cover) to include the most current information possible. These books are valuable because they have stood the test of time, the author took the time to add new information over the years, and they were helpful enough to remain in high demand.

• *Books sponsored or endorsed by a familiar national health organization*. If a well-respected disease-specific organization is involved with the book, it has an added "seal of approval" since the organization won't want to have its name associated with poorly written or inaccurate material. Also, these types of books will often go through several stages of fact-checking and approval processes, which helps ensure a high-quality product. The American Diabetes Association, American Cancer Society, American Lung Association, American Dietetic Association, Arthritis Foundation, American Geriatric Society, and many others have associated themselves with excellent disease-specific books.

• *Signs of research*. Flip through the book and see whether physicians or scientists are quoted, or if reference is made to scientific research that backs up the theory being proposed. (Some of the best books will also list references, resources, and/or bibliographies at the end of each chapter or at the end of the book.) These are signs that the information in the book is supported by sound principles and generally accepted research. If these signs are not there, skip the book and look for one with better backup.

• *Credentials*. Check to see who wrote the book, then judge if that person is capable of writing medical information you can trust. For example, is the writer a medical doctor (an "M.D.")?

That's a good start, but you've got to look further than that. Although we'd like to think that anything written by a medical doctor must be medically accurate, that's not always true. Unfortunately, as with any profession, there are renegades among doctors—those who champion unproved (and sometimes dangerous) disease theories or treatments, or those who become mired in commercialism. If the doctor who wrote the book also lists references, the information in the book is probably good. But what about books that are not written by an M.D.? Should you automatically ignore them? No, but be more wary. If the writer has a Ph.D., look at the author biography to see if you can find out what the Ph.D. is in. Sometimes the advanced degree makes sense, other times it doesn't. A writer with a Ph.D. in nutrition is certainly a reliable source for a nutrition book, but would be a less-respected source for a psychology book. And then there are the medical writers, those who do not have medical degrees but are writing about medical topics. Can you trust them? It depends . . . medical writers are specialists in presenting information in a balanced and easy-to-understand manner, but they need to have their facts straight. Look in the acknowledgments section to see if any medical experts were consulted in the research for the book *and* look to see if references are made to scientific research. If not, skip the book.

• *Necessary information.* Look at the table of contents and the index to see the scope of what is covered in the book. If your needs are not adequately represented, look for a different book. For example, if you are interested in reading about acupuncture, but a book on complementary medicine offers only one general chapter on "Chinese Healing Techniques," skip it and look for a book that addresses your needs more specifically. If, on the other hand, you want to explore alternative medicine to help fight cancer, look for the word *cancer* in the index to see how many pages offer that level of detail. There are so many books covering such a wide variety of topics that you can afford to be choosy about the ones you spend your time and money on.

INSPIRATIONAL

Not all health books provide solid, research-driven information. Inspirational books offer stories of hope to people who are suffering from life-threatening or life-altering diseases. These books can be general, disease-specific, religious, humorous, or even stories of medical miracles.

These are the types of books you'll want to keep on your nightstand for those moments when you wake up in a panic and need to calm your fears before sleeping again—or in your purse or the glove compartment of your car so they are always available, especially if you spend a lot of time waiting in doctors' offices or receive lengthy treatments, such as chemotherapy infusion or dialysis.

There are no rules about what makes "good" or "bad" inspiration. Read the first page or two, then skip to the middle of the book and read another page or two. If the stories or messages "speak" to you, then that's the book for you. There's no such thing as "too inspired," so read as many of these books as you like, and read them as many times as you wish. Many of these books are also available on cassette or compact disc so you can simply plug in and listen! An example of a popular inspirational book is *Chicken Soup for the Soul*, but look beyond the bestseller list, as well, to discover gems—such as Robert Lipsyte's *In the Country of Illness*.

Note: Avoid books that try to "sell" you on a product or treatment plan that they claim will guarantee a cure, or that steer you away from your partnership with your doctor. No matter how well-intentioned they may be, those books have the capacity to be irresponsible and potentially dangerous to your health. If you have any doubts, ask your doctor.

SELF-HELP

There are a broad range of books that patients can use to improve their quality of life or better manage their illness that are not disease-specific or necessarily inspirational. These are books that focus on one specific aspect of the health experience, usually written in a how-to format. For example, there are specialty books that tell you how to talk to your doctor, how to prepare for surgery, how to meditate, or how to eat healthier. Not everyone will feel the need for any or all of these topics, but if they are important to you, certainly add them to your reading list. These types of books tend not to become outdated as quickly as disease-specific books, so the date of publication is not as important. After all, the basics of good nutrition and meditation haven't changed in decades. Some examples are *How to Meditate* by Lawrence LeShan, *Eating Well for Optimum Health* by Andrew Weil, and *Preparing for Surgery* by William Deardorff and John Reeves II.

REFERENCE BOOKS

Medical dictionaries, pharmaceutical drug books, handbooks of diagnostic tests, and other reference books are indispensable for people who are fighting or managing an illness. Their best use is to help you interpret the information you read in your medical file, define specialized words used in journal articles or medical textbooks, or understand instructions or advice from your doctor.

Medical dictionaries: Like a regular dictionary, medical dictionaries define words commonly used in the medical field. There are many to choose from, and they all have their own strengths and weaknesses. Some are written for medical professionals, and therefore use complex words in definitions of even more complex words. Others have photographs or illustrations as visual definitions. Some are simpler but less complete. In a large bookstore, compare dictionaries by choosing three medical terms that you have had trouble understanding from your own experience. Look up the same word in several dictionaries to see how the definitions differ. If you can't understand the definition, choose a different dictionary. Medical dictionaries are updated about every four years, but choose a dictionary based on ease-of-use, not on date. Basic definitions don't change, and unless you have a disorder at the cutting-edge of research, such as AIDS or cancer, and you want highly detailed medical terminology, you won't need the absolute latest version.

Pharmaceutical guides: These are a must for anyone who takes medication, especially if you change or add medications frequently. These guides provide information on drug uses, side effects, proper dosage, drug interactions, and special considerations such as how the drug might affect pregnancy. Again, there are several different drug guides available, each with different strengths. Look up a medication that you are currently taking in different books and see which book presents the information in a way that is convenient and easy for you. Choose the book that you are most comfortable with. New versions of all the books are printed yearly because so many new drugs are approved. As soon as you cannot find in your book a medication you've been prescribed, purchase an updated version.

Other medical reference books: Then there are the books that provide specific information many patients find valuable. There is the *Dictionary of Medical Acronyms & Abbreviations*, which tells what EPTS (existed prior to service), PSA (prostate specific antigen), SCIWORA (spinal cord injury without radiographic abnormality), BHR (basal heart rate), and thousands of other confusing acronyms stand for. There are also books that describe everything you want to know about medical tests— the preparation needed, what the procedure consists of, and what the doctor will be looking for. Although much of this same information can be found in general medical guides, these books give you the information at your fingertips. Whatever your special health needs, there is probably a book to guide you through the process of understanding. Browse through the medical reference section of a large bookstore and see which guides look useful. The goal is to stock your home library with the books you will need to thoroughly understand your medical condition and treatment.

MEDICAL TEXTBOOKS

If your need for detailed disease information still isn't satisfied after reading several consumer books, you may want to try to tackle a medical textbook. Most people won't find the information in a medical textbook helpful . . . it's too detailed, too physiological, and uses nothing but medical jargon. You'll have to read the book with a medical dictionary in your other hand. Another drawback is that medical textbooks aren't carried in most public libraries, so you'll have to purchase them, and they are expensive—most run between $80 and $300. But if you are comfortable reading medicalese and want in-depth information, medical textbooks should be able to help you find answers to even the most detailed questions. The most common medical textbooks are available at large bookstores (such as Barnes and Noble) and general book Internet sites (such as amazon. com). There are also specialized medical book Internet sites that will sell a wider range of professional books and textbooks (such as BookMarc.com, LB.com, and MedBooksNOW.com).

What You Should Know About Libraries

If you haven't set foot in a public library in the last decade, you'll probably be surprised by the changes. The biggest change is that libraries have gone electronic, and the card catalog has gone the way of the dodo bird. No more banks of tiny cards to shuffle through; instead, there are banks of computer monitors that let you type in the title, name of the author, and subject or keyword of the book you are looking for. It will then tell you not only where the book can be found, but whether it is currently on the shelf or checked out.

In addition, nearly every library in the United States has at least one terminal with a connection to the Internet, so if you don't have a computer at home you can do your searching at the library. In many cases, the library has a high-speed connection, so your library search may be quicker than your home search.

Reference librarians will also search special electronic databases to find the exact information you need, giving you online access to hundreds of magazines and journals. A library that once subscribed to three hundred print magazines now has access to more than twelve hundred magazines online. That's good news for the health researcher, but it comes with a downside:

Libraries have less money to spend on books for their collections because they need to spend more money on increasingly expensive journal subscriptions.

While fewer books in the library means you'll have fewer to browse through, you still can borrow just about any book through the interlibrary loan system. If your library doesn't have the book you want, a librarian can request the book from another library for you to borrow. Once you put in your request, the book will reach your library in about one to two weeks, sometimes longer if the book is not easily available. Even the National Library of Medicine participates in this interlibrary loan system, so virtually any health book in existence (and owned by your local library system) can be borrowed. The cost to you: usually nothing, though sometimes there is a small fee. The catch: You need a valid library card. Fortunately, public library cards in the United States are free. Simply go to your local public library with proof of where you live (such as a property tax bill or your driver's license), and they will issue you a card.

If you want to use a library for which you don't have a card, such as the public library in the next county or the library at a public university, you have every right to do so. The only difference is that you will not be able to borrow books (although some might allow borrowing membership for a small fee). Some private libraries, such as those found in private colleges, allow local residents to use their facilities, but it's always a good idea to call in advance to ask about their policy.

Another change you might note in the library is that, in most cases, the atmosphere is different. "Public libraries have opened themselves up," says Daniel O'Connor, Ph.D., M.L.S., associate professor in the Department of Library and Information Science at Rutgers University in New Jersey. "Consumers can expect cooperative, friendly people, especially in the more active libraries. People should feel as though they can approach anybody and ask any question." In other words, there's no reason to feel intimidated by librarians. They are ready, willing, and anxious to help you find what you need. All you have to do is ask.

In fact, it's a good idea to establish an ongoing relationship with one of the reference librarians at your local public library. Introduce yourself and explain your situation. Ask for suggestions about how to search for information in the library and whether the librarian has access to information databases that are usually unavailable to regular citizens. Ask if they could keep an eye out for interesting information for you—librarians often receive reviews of books that will be published in the coming months, so you could get advance notice of them. Later, make sure you say hello whenever you're in the library, and ask if any new books about your disease have come to the librarian's attention. After a while, the librarian will become another partner in your search for health.

But as you develop this partnership, remember that the librarian is there for information only, not for advice. "One of the things that irritates librarians is when the public asks them to provide medical advice," says Dr. O'Connor. "Librarians won't provide legal or medical advice. They can provide people with a lot of medical information on a health topic, but they're not going to assume the role of a health professional. Same is true with pharmaceutical drug information."

Specialty Libraries

Local public libraries are great for convenience, but they may not offer everything you need for a complete health information search. You have three other options: medical school libraries, hospital libraries, and consumer health libraries.

Medical school libraries, obviously, are affiliated with medical schools. Their strength is that they carry more journals than any other source. If you find a valuable journal abstract (see chapter 9), you can find and photocopy the entire article at a medical library. For private universities, call in advance to find out what access you can have to their resources. For public universities, such as the state university system, your tax dollars help support the library, so you should feel comfortable using the facilities. The medical reference librarians there will be more highly trained than the librarian in your average local public library, since they may be accredited by the Academy of Health Information Professionals. This means they have had additional training and have passed testing requirements that make them adept at finding health information. They will be happy to assist you, although there may be a longer wait during some busier academic times. Unless you or a family member actually works for the university, you won't be able to borrow books. (Some universities have a "Friends of the Library" group, which, if you contribute a certain amount of money, will allow you the same access and borrowing privileges as a university member. Ask the librarian at your local medical school library for information about this type of membership.)

Hospital libraries are usually found right inside a large hospital complex. They are mainly used by physicians, nurses, and other staff members, but some allow patients or members of the public to come in to look for journal articles and otherwise use the library. Although the hospital librarian will be happy to point out where a particular book is located or how the copy machine works, he or she generally will not be available to help you search for information. Call in advance to find out if you are able to use their resources.

One of the best-kept secrets in library resources is the consumer health library. These specialized libraries cater to people who want to find out everything they can about their illness. The librarians will listen to your questions and either point you in a direction for finding the information or find the information for you. They loan books, audiotapes and videotapes, photocopy journal articles, find brochures, give contact information for disease associations, and provide just about any other health information function you can think of. They are rather like one-stop shopping for your health information needs.

Where are they? They are usually associated with a hospital, so ask your doctor if your hospital has one. As of this writing, there are one hundred sixty registered consumer health libraries in the United States, and the number is growing. To find the one nearest you, check the online Consumer Health Library Directory at the website for the Consumer and Patient Health Information Section (CAPHIS) of the Medical Library Association (http://caphis.njc.org/Directory/Intro.html).

What makes these libraries such a treasure is that some of them are philanthropically funded, and all have the goal of disseminating health information to the average consumer. This means that in many cases you don't need to go to a consumer health library in your neighborhood to take advantage of it; many will accept questions and information requests over the telephone or by e-mail, and then send you the information, often free of charge, although some may charge a small fee for postage or photocopying. These libraries are a valuable resource for anyone but can be a godsend for those who are so ill that they cannot conduct an information search on their own.

One such consumer health library is the Community Health Resource Library, part of the Geisinger Medical Center in Danville, Pennsylvania. "We wanted to provide a place where people could come to find quality information, so they could make informed decisions about their health and lifestyle," says Valerie Gross, M.L.S., the librarian and codeveloper of the program. "What the consumer health library does is provide a relaxed atmosphere where people can just come, sit down, talk to the librarian, and ask questions. The librarian can go through the collection and pull out resources, books and videotapes, do a literature search, then give that information to the person."

Consumer health librarians have access to specialized health information databases that they will search for the patient, and often have a connection with a medical school or hospital library that cooperates in providing more clinical and technical information.

The Geisinger consumer health library services are available to anyone, as are those of many other consumer health libraries. "I'll take an information request from anyone across the country," says Ms. Gross. "They can call, fax, or e-mail me, and if they are more than an hour from the center, I'll get all the information then mail it to them free of charge. The farthest I've sent information was to Alaska."

The creation of consumer health libraries is becoming a national trend, and for good reason. They can provide a guiding hand in those rough initial days after a diagnosis, as well as long-term lifestyle information for diseases that need to be managed. "We get a lot of people who are coming right out of a doctor's office, they've just been diagnosed with something, and they are upset," says Ms. Gross. "This is a really good place to start because we have some easy-to-understand information on a lot of different conditions. I think having someplace somebody can come, take a really deep breath, find out what the condition is, really can help dispel fear." [The Community Health Resource Library can be reached at 570-271-5638, or visit their website at http://www.geisinger.org/patient/health info/comm.htm for more information. Other consumer health libraries and their contact information are available from the Medical Library Association at http://caphis.njc.org/Directory/ Intro.html.]

▶ ACTION PLAN—USING BOOKS AS RESOURCES

1. Be choosy about the health books you read. Make sure they are relatively current, have the information you need, and are written by reputable sources that have backup in the form of listed resources, reviewers, or scientific research.

2. Start a home library. The basics: a general medical guide and a medical dictionary. Other guides, how-to books, specialty books, and inspirational books can be added at your discretion.

3. Partner with your local librarian. Obtain a library card and take advantage of the interlibrary loan system to borrow just about any health book.

4. Locate a consumer health library to help you gather medical information. It can either be one near you, or one that is willing to find and ship information to you.
5. Note important or inspiring books in the journal portion of your Personal Health Log, especially if the book was borrowed. If you own the book, tag pages with information you might want to return to with Post-It notes.

6. Mass Media: Newspapers, Television, Radio

Value as a health information source: ★ ☆ ☆ ☆

Effort required: ★ ☆ ☆ ☆

Accessibility: ★ ★ ★ ★

Good for: Getting initial information about treatment or drug breakthroughs. Always requires further investigation.

THERE are certain health facts we used to feel pretty confident about: A high-fiber diet prevents colon cancer. The lower your cholesterol level, the better. Avoid eggs at all costs. Simple. No-brainers.

Except for one thing: The media reported, rather forcefully, that medical studies found exactly the opposite. From bold headlines and sincere correspondents, we learned that:

- A high-fiber diet does not prevent colon cancer.
- Low cholesterol leads to greater risk of stroke.
- Eating as much as one egg a day doesn't hurt you.

In each case, there was more to the story than most mass-media reports were able to convey. If you only read the headline, skimmed the article, or listened to the report while feeding the dog, it would be easy to miss the critical details. In fact, the conclusions bulleted above are, at least in part, wrong. Why? We'll get back to that. First, a little background. . . .

How a Medical Finding Makes the News

Anyone who reads the newspaper, watches TV, or listens to the radio can't help but feel confused, frustrated, and angered by the contradictory health information we are bombarded with every day. The result is a collective wish that all those doctors and researchers would just make up their minds. After all, how many times can we have trusted medical beliefs shattered before we decide not to believe anything?

First of all, don't blame the scientists. Medical researchers spend their lives doing studies on a small, well-defined portion of a larger problem with the hope that some day, if they are both diligent and lucky, they will help develop a cure for a disease. When they finish a study, they analyze the results using statistics. If the results are important to the scientific community, the researchers write up an article describing what they found and submit it to a medical journal with the hope that it will be published. (Researchers have a lot to gain by publishing articles, including promotions, raises, grant funding, and tenure at a university.)

Hundreds of studies are published every day. Some of the larger, more prestigious journals—such as the *New England Journal of Medicine, The Lancet, Journal of the American Medical Association*, and the *British Journal of Medicine*—have their more interesting articles summarized by news service organizations, such as Reuters (pronounced ROY-ters) or Associated Press (AP). These organizations feed ready-made news stories to newspapers and television and radio stations throughout the country. If you look just beneath the headline of news stories in your local paper, chances are you'll see the author's name, often followed by "Of the Associated Press" or "Reuters."

Do the AP and Reuters summarize *every* journal article that's published? Hardly. There wouldn't be enough time in the day or space in the newspaper. They choose the articles that are the most significant and/or interesting. Then, the local newspaper or television news station has to choose from among all the news-feed stories they receive. Now, imagine for a moment that you are in charge of the health section of your local newspaper, and you have a choice of printing an article based on one of the following studies. Which would you choose? (These are actual studies that were reported on the same day in 1999.)

A. A study that found that using radiofrequency energy can reduce tongue volume and therefore help people with sleep apnea.
B. A report about how the drugs Mirapex (pramipexole) and Requip (ropinirole), used to treat Parkinson's disease, caused eight men to fall asleep uncontrollably.
C. A study that found that cigar smokers are more likely to develop cancer and heart disease than nonsmokers.

If you chose "a" or "b," chances are you know someone who suffers from sleep apnea or Parkinson's disease. If you chose "c," then you earn the title "newshound." Cigar smoking became a popular fad in the 1990s. Movie stars smoke cigars, TV programs depict women smoking cigars, and cigar-bars have cropped up in every major city. Choice "c" is exciting . . . it's "sexy" . . . it will get people reading. That doesn't mean choices "a" or "b" aren't important. In fact, they are potentially very important to people diagnosed with sleep apnea or Parkinson's disease. They just aren't as entertaining or as likely to raise the ratings of a TV news show. Therefore, you are less likely to hear about them.

So every time you read or hear or see a health report, remember what you're getting—the prechosen story of the day, glamorized and trumped up to be more important than it is. It gets our attention. And these days, mass media tend to be more concerned with profit and ratings than providing good, honest reporting on solid medical research.

How to Understand a Media Report

This doesn't mean you have to stop reading the newspaper or listening to your favorite news show. You just have to know how to interpret the news you get. That way, you won't feel disappointed when you find out that the story was more sizzle than steak.

DON'T MAKE DECISIONS
BASED ON A SINGLE STUDY

Medical truth is like a jigsaw puzzle, and each study or finding is just one piece of the puzzle. No single piece can give you the whole picture. Only when enough individual pieces are joined together will the picture begin to make sense.

Medical science is a process of continual discovery. What we now know to be true has been built on observations and experiments conducted over many years. Each study you read about is only a small piece of a growing body of knowledge. That one small piece may contain valuable information, but it only makes sense when you look at it in context with all the other research.

So when you hear about a new research report, ask yourself how this new information fits with information you've read in the past. Does this information fit with what you already understand about your disease, or does it contradict what you know? If it fits, then there's nothing more you need to do. But if it seems to be a substantial change in what you know, ask your doctor how this new information relates to you and your specific condition. Does the article recommend that you change your behavior in any way due to this finding? If so, speak with your doctor first. Don't change your treatment due to a single article or news report.

MAKE SURE YOU HAVE THE FULL STORY

Media coverage of a medical news story can be superficial and sensational. Their job is to catch your attention, give you the basic facts, and move on to the next story. Needless to say, there is not much time for analysis of the "big picture," and the headlines can often be startling or unsettling.

Maurie Markman, M.D., director of the Cleveland Clinic Taussig Cancer Center, is concerned with the confusion news stories can create. "When you're dealing with something like cancer, the topic is extraordinarily complicated," says Dr. Markman. Misinformation and oversimplified information can play on the emotions of patients, creating panic, unrealistic expectations, or discouragement. Scientists work for years forming a small part of that puzzle, and produce a detailed report, "and it's then written up by a reporter who's trying to simplify it for a thirty-second sound bite on the news," Dr. Markman continues. "Just today, on [a popular TV news show] there was a report about an ultrasound test and how effective it is potentially to find early-stage ovarian cancer. Total, complete, absolute misinformation, but do you know how many women are going to go out there now and want ultrasounds from their gynecologists? We've had dozens of calls here already, women asking if they can have this test. Would I say the reporters have done the best they can do? It's an extraordinarily complicated topic, and it's been presented in a completely inappropriate way. Has damage been done? Hard to say, because tomorrow the story will be gone, and they'll be on to their next sensational topic."

So before jumping to conclusions, or calling your doctor, or believing the news report, wait to hear the whole story, especially if the news seems too good (or too bad) to be true. Don't lose hope or feel distressed based on a single study report. Watch for follow-up stories that may provide a more complete analysis, or, if the report was based on a journal article (and it will usually say so somewhere in the report), find and read the whole article. If you find yourself so worried that you are unable to sleep, ask your doctor to explain what the story might mean for *you*.

EVALUATE THE INFORMATION GIVEN

There are certain guideposts in every story that can tell you how valuable a particular study may be. Some of the most important:

• *Is the information based on experimental data or anecdotes?* While stories of patients who recovered from a disease after a particular treatment are intriguing, they cannot be considered part of medical knowledge until a scientific study is conducted. Anecdotes without experimental data to back them up are not reliable sources of medical information.

• *Where was the study conducted?* In general, studies conducted by government institutions (such as the National Cancer Institute or the Food and Drug Administration) or major universities and medical schools will be well-designed and appropriately interpreted. These institutions have strict experimental protocols they must follow and have the resources to get the job done right. Be wary of studies that come from pharmaceutical companies or other organizations, since the results may be biased. Also, studies conducted in other countries may be accurate, but the outcomes may not be applicable to the American public, since diets, environmental factors, pollution levels, and other differences may alter the results.

• *Did an outside agency fund the study?* Studies funded by manufacturers or conducted by insider industry groups may be biased. For example, it is unlikely that research funded by the tobacco companies will find that smoking is harmful.

• *Was this a preliminary study?* If it is, it usually says so. If so, it should be given less weight than more definitive studies or follow-ups.

• *Did the study use human subjects or animals?* Rats are not humans, and humans are not rats. Although animal studies are the first step all scientists need to take before conducting human studies and are the basis of most medical discoveries, don't try to apply the results of studies on animals to your own condition. Drugs and treatments that work perfectly well in rodents may have no effect in humans, or they may be the next big breakthrough. There are no guarantees. Under the best circumstances, applying animal cures to human disease will take years of additional research. Look at reports of animal research with interest and cautious long-term optimism.

• *Who participated in the study?* The types of human subjects used in the study may make the results less useful for you. For example, results of a study that included only men may not be applicable to women, and a study that included only Caucasian subjects may not be applicable to African Americans. The more general the type of subjects used, the more you'll be able to generalize the results. (On the other hand, if you're a man, a study done only on men is likely to be even more applicable to you than a study done using both men and women.)

• *How many subjects were used?* In general, the greater the number of people tested, the more reliable the information. If the study looked at 12 people, the results will be less reliable than one that looked at 120 people, and that will be less reliable than a study that looked at 1,200 or 12,000 people. A good rule of thumb: Dismiss any study that used fewer than 100 people. If the results of a smaller study were remarkable, the research will be repeated using more subjects.

UNDERSTAND THE EXACT NATURE
OF THE QUESTION

Medical research tackles big questions by breaking them down into a series of smaller questions. This microscopic focus results in small, limited findings. If researchers report that they studied the effects of monounsaturated fats on circulating levels of cholesterol one hour after a meal, that's exactly what they looked at. They did not look at *all* fats, or at risk of heart attack, or at generally high cholesterol readings.

Examine the purpose and details of the study carefully. Don't generalize the findings more broadly than what was intended. Look for the scientist's analysis of how this specific study fits in with the broader picture.

CORRELATION DOES NOT EQUAL CAUSATION

Scientists don't use the word "cause" lightly, as in "broken bones *cause* pain." Instead, they often talk about correlations or relationships among variables, meaning things that occur together. It's valuable to remember that just because two things happen simultaneously doesn't mean that one *causes* the other. For example, scientists have found that low socioeconomic status is related to a higher risk of ulcers, but being poor doesn't *cause* ulcers. Rather, low socioeconomic status is related to many other factors, such as a poor diet, greater stress, and perhaps a greater exposure to disease . . . any or all (or none) of which may be the true cause of ulcers.

On the other hand, correlations and relationships are important, too. For example, it is known that obesity is *related* to many disorders, including increased risk of diabetes and heart disease. It would be foolish to disregard this information just because a *causal* relationship has not been determined.

Strong correlational relationships are often linked to a common cause, even if we don't yet know what it is. Don't deny or ignore a relationship just because it isn't a defined *cause*, but don't assume causation from a correlation.

REACT CAUTIOUSLY

Every now and then, newspapers publish articles about cars that run on electricity instead of gasoline. The first time you read about them, you didn't run out to buy one. Even if they had been available, you would have wanted to see how durable they were, how much they cost to run and how fast they could go before you'd fork over your money.

The next time you read or hear about a new medical study, disease treatment, or diet book, take time to evaluate it. Watch for an analysis by medical experts to tell you how this study fits in with what is already known. Use the information judiciously, piece by piece, to build your own understanding of the big picture. Again, if you are left feeling uncomfortable or confused, always speak with your doctor about your concerns.

One of the more troubling trends in recent years is the use of "teasers" by television news programs. You know how it goes . . . you're watching your favorite television show during prime time, and during a commercial the local news team tells you, "Doctors say cancer cure just around the corner," or "This popular drug could kill you," followed by a promise of more information if you "tune in at eleven for more details." In a few circumstances, the information may be an important public health announcement that may immediately have an impact on your life, such as a recall of a certain food that was found to be tainted. But for the most part, the information is just another highly sensationalized news story, except you've now had a couple of hours since the teaser to either get really excited or really worried about the news. Tune in the news, but learn to tune out the teasers.

Now, with that background, we can get back to the stories cited at the beginning of this chapter. Using the guidelines outlined above, we can see how the headlines could be found to be misleading or just plain wrong. How?

• *A high-fiber diet does not prevent colon cancer.* In fact, this study, reported in January 1999 in the *New England Journal of Medicine* by researchers from Harvard Medical School, never looked at people eating a high-fiber diet. The average American eats about 15 grams of fiber a day. "High fiber" is defined by doctors and dietitians as *at least* 30 grams per day, but possibly up to 50 grams per day (finding this fact would have required additional research). The women in the study (yes, only women were used, so men should have been wary about this study right from the start) who supposedly were eating a "high-fiber" diet were eating only 25 grams of fiber a day. That's not high fiber! The study demonstrated, then, that colon cancer wasn't prevented if women ate a diet with low or medium amounts of fiber. How many people were fooled into giving up their bran cereal because of misleading headlines? It may be true that fiber doesn't prevent colon cancer, but no single study should be considered definitive proof.

• *Low cholesterol leads to greater risk of stroke.* Read this article from researchers in Japan carefully and you'll discover two very important caveats that got glossed over in most media accounts: (1) The risk was higher for hemorrhagic stroke only—in which there is bleeding in the brain—and (2) cholesterol levels were abnormally low. Most cholesterol is made in our own bodies.

Even if you completely stop consuming any cholesterol, you still won't get down to levels as low as the people in this study. It is likely that the strokes were not *caused* by low cholesterol but were simply correlated with it. Further, the type of stroke most of us need to worry about is ischemic stroke, in which blood vessels become blocked. The vast majority of all strokes—about 85 percent—are ischemic. And one of the risk factors for ischemic stroke is—you guessed it—high cholesterol. People who read this story quickly might have been tempted to throw their old low-cholesterol diets out the window, leaving themselves open to the much greater risk of ischemic stroke.

• *Eating up to one egg each day doesn't hurt you.* A closer look at the details showed that the people in the study, reported in April 1999 by researchers from Harvard University, were healthy people with no history of heart disease or high cholesterol. This means that if you already have heart disease or cholesterol, doctors still don't know if eggs (notoriously high in cholesterol) will hurt you.

▶ ACTION PLAN—BE WARY OF INFORMATION FROM MASS MEDIA

1. Don't change your behavior or get worried and upset because of a single study or medical news report.
2. Look for the details. Many studies can be disregarded as unimportant to your personal situation if you read carefully.
3. Use news reports as a starting point for further research. If a report looks promising, read the original journal article (see chapter 9). That way, you're not getting someone else's summary; you're getting the information straight from the doctors involved.
4. If an article seems appropriate for your condition, cut it out and put it in your Personal Health Log. Write down your observations and questions. If you can't answer the questions after you gather more information, ask your doctor about it.

FURTHER IDEAS: WHEN JOURNALISTS TAKE THEIR TIME

Time is a journalist's best tool for health reporting. Coverage and accuracy suffer when there is pressure to have a story begun and finished within an afternoon or even an hour. Good health writing needs perspective, which can be offered only by taking one's time and by listening to various experts who might have differing opinions about how important or unimportant a given "medical breakthrough" may be. In today's fast-moving media marketplace, time is in short supply.

Fortunately, not all media reports are quick sound bites or knee-jerk news stories. "Dateline," "20/20," "48 Hours," and other long-format television news shows air nightly, and many times the topic of the segment is health-related. Also, health is beginning to dominate certain television channels, such as Discovery Health and TLC, The Learning Channel. Although most of the programs are highly accurate and well-researched, watch them with skepticism. As you watch, closely observe:

- *The quality of physicians interviewed.* If the doctors interviewed are from Harvard Medical School, Mount Sinai Medical Center, the Mayo Clinic, Duke University, or other highly rated and well-respected medical establishments, chances are the information is worth listening to.
- *The qualifications of others who are interviewed.* As a comparison, in the past, dangerous exercise routines and diets have been promoted by some celebrities who happened to be fit. While celebrities make terrific spokespersons, they have not had the years of training required to understand body kinetics, metabolism, and physiology. The same is true of all other aspects of health. Make sure you understand the qualifications of the person being interviewed and ignore unsubstantiated advice.
- *If this is a balanced presentation.* Does the program show more than just a single perspective? If not, there may be bias in the reporting.

• *If there is a tone of evangelism.* No therapy, diet, exercise routine, or anything else is right for all people. Be wary of individuals who sound as if they are giving a blanket health recommendation.

Some newspapers offer medical articles that are more in-depth. When reporters are allowed to do their own investigative searches or take the time to consider the ramifications of new research, the results can be wonderful. You'll know these articles right away because the quality strikes you as a breath of fresh air in the otherwise plodding news-feed quickies. These articles present a full and considered story, complete with comments by several physicians and experts. There will be no "AP" or "Reuters" after the author's name. The best health journalists are associated with the best newspapers in the country, especially large-city newspapers such as the *New York Times* and the *Washington Post.*

Even better are the rare times a newspaper has a dedicated health columnist who writes review articles for the average person. For example, the *New York Times* offers a weekly column called "Personal Health" by Jane E. Brody in which topics are covered in a well-rounded way. Ms. Brody dispels myths and informs readers about a wide range of health topics, including atrial fibrillation, cholesterol, dieting, cancer, breast feeding, bereavement, and alternative medicine. Each column discusses a single health topic in engaging, easy-to-understand language, all supported by references to research and interviews with prominent physicians. Her columns are considered the gold standard for consumer health writing. If your newspaper has a similar columnist, consider yourself lucky. If not, you can certainly check out "Personal Health" every Tuesday in the Health section of the *New York Times,* which is available free online at www.nytimes.com.

Final Tips: Finding Mass Media Reports

Most of the time, you'll only want to use a mass media report for background information before starting a more detailed search of medical journals. However, there may be times you'll want to locate a specific article or get the transcript of a show, perhaps because you forgot the name of a doctor who was quoted.

This is not always an easy task. (For the future, it is highly recommended that you write everything down the first time you hear it.)

NEWSPAPERS

If the article you need was from Reuters and published in 1995 or later, you're in luck. The Reuters website (http://www.reuters health.com) allows consumers to search their archives online. (See chapter 8 for more information about how to search and access sites on the Internet.)

Associated Press articles can be found via the Lexis-Nexis index. This is an archive of thousands of different printed sources, including *USA Today*, the *Washington Post*, and numerous local newspapers. You can check to see if the newspaper you are looking for is a source by searching the Lexis-Nexis website (http://www.lexis-nexis.com/lncc/sources). If so, the next trick is locating a place where you can access Lexis-Nexis. Larger libraries may subscribe to Lexis-Nexis, but since the service is rather expensive, smaller libraries won't have it. Check with your local reference librarian to see if Lexis-Nexis is available. If not, check the libraries of local colleges and universities. They may allow nonstudents free access, but some will charge a processing fee.

The *New York Times* has its own index for locating previously published articles. Check your local library to see if they carry it. You'll need to know the year the article was published—and be prepared for a long, tedious search. If the article was published within the past year, the *New York Times* offers an online searchable archive (http://archives.nytimes.com/archives). You can search for free, but there is a small charge, currently $2.50, to download the article.

Many other newspapers also have searchable, downloadable archives online. Search "newspapers" on the Internet for a complete list. All allow you to search for no charge, but registration and a fee is required to read the article. The number of years archived varies. Some of the larger sites are:

Atlanta Journal-Constitution
  (http://www.accessatlanta.com/partners/ajc)
Baltimore Sun
  (http://www.sunspot.net)
Boston Globe
  (http://www.boston.com/globe)
Chicago Tribune
  (http://chicagotribune.com)
Detroit Free Press
  (http://www.freep.com)
Los Angeles Times
  (http://www.latimes.com)
Miami Herald
  (http://www.herald.com)
USA Today
  (http://www.usatoday.com)
Washington Post
  (http://www.washingtonpost.com)

TELEVISION/RADIO

Your best bet for tracking down television or radio transcripts or tapes is to call the station directly. Let them know the specific show, date, and time of the program you need, and they will either place the order for you or tell you the company that handles the transcript service for them. (The company with the largest database devoted to broadcast transcripts is Burrelle's Information Services, which can be contacted at 1-800-777-8398 or through the Internet at www.burrelles.com.) There is always a fee, usually $5 to $7 for written transcripts, and about $29.95 plus shipping for videotapes. Be forewarned: If you later discover you ordered the wrong show, there are no refunds.

Many stations and television shows have Internet sites that often contain show information, or, as in the case of National Public Radio (http://www.npr.org), the full audio that can be played over your computer's speakers. Search "television networks," "radio stations," or the specific name—such as "Discovery Channel" or "Rosie O'Donnell Show"—to find an existing website.

7. Government

Value as a health information source: ★ ★ ★ ★

Effort required: ★ ★ ☆ ☆

Accessibility: ★ ★ ★ ☆

Good for: Accurate information often presented in an easy-to-understand manner. Take advantage of these sources.

THE U.S. government offers some of the best consumer-friendly health information anywhere. Surprised? Many people are, especially since government documents are stereotypically thought to be inaccessible and filled with confusing double-speak. But when it comes to health, the government has made a strong commitment to providing top-notch brochures, web-sites, booklets, and other health-related material. Their work is fast becoming the standard and a resource for other health information providers, such as Internet health websites and newsletters.

The strength of the information comes from the caliber of the people who work for the government. These agencies employ some of the best scientists in the world, and competition for positions can be fierce. The U.S. government takes its mandate to educate the public seriously. Their information is considered to be highly accurate and reliable by just about everyone, and it is often cited and used by other health sources. For example, many for-profit consumer health websites link to U.S. government sites because its reputation for high-quality health information is beyond reproach. Government agencies have been attempting to make their information more easily accessible and readable. They excel in providing clear explanation of general information, statistics, and referrals to other organizations and information sources, but more detailed (and complex) information about specific diseases and treatments can often be found as well.

The main weaknesses of government information are that the overall structure of the health agencies can be confusing and frustrating to navigate, and that the amount of information they generate is so vast that it can quickly become overwhelming, especially if you have to wade through the "official" information in a search for consumer information. For example, a simple search for a particular drug name on the FDA website will return pages upon pages of product-labeling guidelines, applications from the pharmaceutical company seeking approval, transcripts from the drug approval process meetings, announcements of the approval, labeling changes . . . and consumer health articles.

But because so much information in government sources is being generated, much of it is not updated regularly. Since most government documents are dated or report when the documents were last updated, it's usually easy to know how current they are. Look for update statements and factor that information into your reading. Documents that have not been updated in six months may contain obsolete information, especially if they're about medications and treatment procedures. (As with books and other information sources, basic information about disease processes and descriptions don't go out of date as quickly, and can usually be trusted, even if the document is many years old.)

Many government websites offer information geared to two different audiences, with one section for the general public and another for physicians and professionals. (These usually have separate links on the agency's homepage.) Start by reading the information designed for patients and the public first. These sections will explain disease processes, physiology, diagnosis, treatments, and other information in language most people can understand easily. If you want more information after reading those sections, check out the information written for physicians and professionals. (There are no Internet police to stop you from looking at these "professional" sections!) They will be more difficult to understand, but the information will be more detailed and extensive. If you have a good basic understanding of your disorder, you should be able to read through these advanced sections successfully with the help of a medical dictionary.

Finding Government Information

Most consumer health information disseminated by the government comes from the Department of Health and Human Services (HHS). Within this department are the various centers, administrations, and institutes that do research, make policy, and provide health and medical information to consumers, physicians, and other health professionals. Some other departments, such as the Environmental Protection Agency (EPA) and the Department of Agriculture (USDA), also provide some health information.

The best way to access the information from these agencies is through the Internet. But if you don't have access to the Internet, many of the individual agencies and institutes also have a consumer information telephone line, and some offer a phone-in fax service that allows you to call up, order a document by number, and receive it over your personal fax machine. (Document numbers are typically listed in a special "document booklet" you must order in advance by calling the phone-in fax number for that agency and following the directions given.) At the very least, you can call up the main telephone number for each of the agencies and ask to be connected to the public affairs or communications office. (Telephone numbers for federal health information centers and clearinghouses can be found on the website for the National Health Information Center at http://www.health.gov/nhic.)

The U.S. government has several outstanding Internet search tools, including *healthfinder*™ (http://www.healthfinder.gov), the National Women's Health Information Center (http://www.4women.gov), and MEDLINEplus (http://medlineplus.nlm.nih.gov/medlineplus), which links to reviewed and approved health information from government and outside sources. These sites are described in more detail in chapter 8.

Three agencies generate the bulk of the government information you'll find most useful: the National Institutes of Health (NIH), the Centers for Disease Control and Prevention (CDC), and the Food and Drug Administration (FDA). Each agency has very specific functions and scope of information.

National Institutes of Health (NIH)

The NIH is the principal biomedical research agency of the government. It conducts and funds medical research on a wide variety of disease topics, with the goals of improving medical knowledge and determining the future direction of medical treatments and disease prevention. The NIH Internet homepage is at http://www.nih.gov.

The NIH is made up of individual institutes that focus on particular diseases or research areas, each with its own website. On many sites, a Spanish-language option is available. Most also have a telephone help line or fax line through which documents can be ordered.

The main NIH website offers quite a bit of information. Under "Health Information," the NIH links to sections that allow you to order full-text publications; look up all NIH and other toll-free health information telephone lines; read about special programs in rare diseases, women's health, AIDS research, and other topics; link to MEDLINEplus; and find information about clinical trials (see chapter 16).

But the bulk of the information is provided by the individual institutes. No matter which disease or condition you are investigating, chances are the NIH has information available. There are currently four ways of finding NIH information:

1. Through the *healthfinder* Internet site, which links directly to consumer-oriented NIH articles that fit the search parameters.
2. Through a general NIH Internet search, using the "search" function found on the NIH homepage. This can turn up a broad range of articles or documents, many of which may be irrelevant. If want to see absolutely everything the NIH has printed about your topic, and you don't mind sifting through pages of Internet documents, this type of search may be the best.
3. Through the NIH Health Information Index (on the Internet). From the NIH homepage, go to the "Health Information" section, then click on the "NIH Health Information Index" link. This site allows you to choose or browse topics, and then takes you to the specific institute that contains information on that subject. For example, if you are not sure which institute would contain information on abdominal aortic aneurysms, look for "aneurysm" under the "A-E" list. The link to the appropriate institute will be provided (in this case, the National Heart, Lung and Blood Institute), along with a telephone number for that institute if you prefer to call. (*Note:* The area code for all NIH telephone numbers is 301.) This site will not direct you to specific articles or research information, just to the appropriate institute. You'll have to do another search there. Your search may or may not turn up a document—just because this search option leads you to an appropriate institution doesn't mean that there will be any articles available, just that that is the appropriate agency to contact.
4. Through the specific institute that covers the condition you're interested in. If you know which institute has information on your disorder, go to that institute's website and do a search there, or call their information telephone or fax

numbers. This is the quickest way to get to focused information about your condition.

NIH institutes that provide consumer disease and disease prevention information are:

National Cancer Institute (NCI): NCI provides cutting edge information on all types of cancer, including causes, prevention, detection, diagnosis, treatment, and control. There are huge amounts of information available on the website, including full-text versions of their booklets (under "publications"). Anyone can call the NCI's Cancer Information Service confidential, toll-free telephone help line. It is staffed with information specialists who can help you find information about any of your cancer concerns free of charge.
   Website: http://www.nci.nih.gov
   Telephone information: 1-800-4-CANCER (1-800-422-6237)
      1-800-332-8615 (TTY)

National Institute of Diabetes and Digestive and Kidney Diseases (NIDDK): NIDDK provides extensive information about diabetes; endocrine and metabolic diseases; digestive diseases and nutrition; and kidney, urologic, and hematologic diseases.
   Website: http://www.niddk.nih.gov
   Telephone: 301-654-3327 (National Diabetes Information
      Clearinghouse)
      301-654-3810 (National Digestive Diseases Information
      Clearinghouse)

National Heart, Lung, and Blood Institute (NHLBI): NHLBI provides information on diseases of the heart, blood vessels, lungs, and blood and on transfusion medicine. These include all heart disorders, asthma, Raynaud's phenomenon, hemophilia, sickle cell anemia, hypertension, chronic obstructive pulmonary disease, cystic fibrosis, insomnia, and narcolepsy.
   Website: http://www.nhlbi.nih.gov
   Telephone: 301-592-8573

National Institute of Dental and Craniofacial Research (NIDCR): NIDCR provides information about infectious and inherited craniofacial-oral-dental diseases and disorders, such as achrondroplasia, dentinogenesis imperfecta, and Prader-Willi syndrome.

Website: http://www.nidcr.nih.gov

Telephone: 301-402-7364 (National Oral Health Information Clearinghouse)

National Institute of Neurological Disorders and Stroke (NINDS): NINDS provides information about the causes, prevention, diagnosis, and treatment of more than six hundred nervous system disorders, including stroke, epilepsy, multiple sclerosis, Parkinson's disease, head and spinal cord injury, Alzheimer's disease, and brain tumors.

Website: http://www.ninds.nih.gov

Telephone: 1-800-352-9424

National Institute of Allergy and Infectious Diseases (NIAID): NIAID provides information on many infectious, immunologic, and allergic diseases, including tuberculosis, AIDS, chronic fatigue syndrome, Lyme disease, hepatitis, colds, and influenza. Full-text publications available online.

Website: http://www.niaid.nih.gov

Telephone: 301-402-1663

National Eye Institute (NEI): NEI provides information about blinding eye diseases, visual disorders, mechanisms of visual function, preservation of sight, and the special health problems and requirements of the blind. Go to the "Public and Patients" section for information on glaucoma, macular degeneration, diabetic retinopathy, cataracts, histoplasmosis, and other eye disorders. This site also provides information on financial aid and other assistance programs for people with eye disorders, how to order large-print publications, and a form for submitting a question to the NEI via e-mail.

Website: http://www.nei.nih.gov
Telephone: 301-496-5248

National Institute of Arthritis and Musculoskeletal and Skin Diseases (NIAMS): NIAMS provides limited information about the causes, treatment, and prevention of arthritis and musculoskeletal and skin diseases, including atopic dermatitis, avascular necrosis, fibromyalgia, gout, psoriasis, Marfan syndrome, vitiligo, lupus, and all forms of arthritis.

Website: http://www.nih.gov/niams
Telephone: 301-495-4484
  877-22-NIAMS (toll free)
  301-565-2966 (TTY)

National Institute on Deafness and Other Communication Disorders (NIDCD): NIDCD provides information on diseases and disorders of hearing, balance, smell, taste, voice, speech, and language.

Website: http://www.nidcd.nih.gov
Telephone: 1-800-241-1044
  1-800-241-1055 (TTY)

National Institute of Mental Health (NIMH): NIMH provides information about mental illnesses, including bipolar disorder, depression, phobias, obsessive-compulsive disorder, schizophrenia, and post-traumatic stress disorder.

Website: http://www.nimh.nih.gov
Telephone: 301-443-4513 (general)
  1-888-8-ANXIETY (1-888-826-9438—for anxiety)
  1-800-421-4211 (for depression)
  1-800-64-PANIC (1-800-647-2642—for panic)

National Institute on Drug Abuse (NIDA): NIDA provides information about drugs of abuse, guides for parents, and treatment information. Also provides links and resources. Greatest strength is the information hotlines.

Website: http://www.drugabuse.gov
Telephone: 1-800-729-6686 (National Clearinghouse for
    Alcohol and Drug Information)
InfoFax: 1-888-NIH-NIDA (1-888-644-6432)
    1-888-TTY-NIDA (1-888-889-6432—TTY)

National Institute on Alcohol Abuse and Alcoholism (NIAAA):
NIAAA provides information on the treatment and preven-
tion of alcoholism and alcohol-related disorders. Website has
full-text booklets about alcoholism and how to cut down on
drinking, as well as other resources to contact.
Website: http://www.niaaa.nih.gov
Telephone: 1-800-729-6686 (National Clearinghouse for
    Alcohol and Drug Information)
InfoFax: 1-888-NIH-NIDA (1-888-644-6432)
    1-888-TTY-NIDA (1-888-889-6432—TTY)

Centers for Disease
Control and Prevention (CDC)

The CDC is the agency in charge of protecting the public
health through the prevention and control of diseases and
other preventable conditions. This is the "sexy" health agency,
the one with the "virus hunters" wearing Level 4 Biohazard
protection suits, the one they write novels and movies about.
CDC information is available by telephone at 1-800-311-3435
or 404-639-3534, or on the Internet at http://www.cdc.gov.

For the consumer, the CDC's strength is in providing information on disease prevention. Although this may not seem
important if you already have a disease, it may be worthwhile
reading up on prevention to see if there is anything you could
be doing that might help prevent a recurrence or a worsening
of the disorder.

The CDC also provides basic information about exotic diseases (everything from African sleeping sickness to West Nile
encephalitis), travelers' health, and prevention of more common

transmissible diseases such as HIV, AIDS, influenza, tuberculosis, and hepatitis. To access this information, click on the link to "Health Topics A to Z" on the homepage, then search list for the condition in which you are interested.

The section on travelers' health is particularly noteworthy. It provides information on health hazards by travel destination, recommendations on how to avoid getting sick while traveling, advice for special needs travelers (those with disabilities or HIV, and women who are pregnant or breastfeeding), and travel vaccinations. There is a special Travelers' Health Hotline that can be reached by calling 877-FYI-TRIP. You can order information to be sent to you or you can listen to recorded information about specific diseases. (All this information is available on the website, so if you have Internet access, that is your best bet.)

If you go to the CDC Internet site, you'll see many references to the CDC's magazine, *Morbidity and Mortality Weekly Report* (*MMWR*). This publication prints information about the incidence and prevalence of diseases and their effects—basically, how many people have it, how many people die of it, where are the outbreaks, and other statistical facts. If this is interesting to you, feel free to search past issues of the *MMWR* online. But most people won't have any need for this information.

Food and Drug Administration (FDA)

The FDA has a mission to protect the consumer by ensuring that food is safe, pure, and wholesome; that electronic products that emit radiation are safe; and that drugs and medical devices are safe and effective. This is the organization that approves new medications and medical devices, regulates pharmaceuticals, and provides guidance about food safety and nutrition. If you have a question about a drug or a medical device, this is the place to go. Its website is located at http://www.fda.gov, and the toll-free telephone number is 1-888-INFO-FDA (1-888-463-6332).

Unfortunately, the FDA website is the least consumer-friendly of all the government health information sites. This is partly due to the fact that the FDA serves a number of different populations—not only patients and consumers but physicians who need information, physicians who need to report medication problems, dietitians, medical device manufacturers, and people from the pharmaceutical industry. The benefit of this diversity of information is that you have access to the same documents as industry professionals. But you'll need to be persistent and patient to locate the information you want.

From the FDA homepage, you can either search the entire FDA site by keyword or go to any of the subareas of the FDA. Most helpful are the Center for Drug Evaluation and Research (click "Drugs" on the homepage), the Center for Food Safety and Applied Nutrition (click "Food" on the homepage), or the Center for Devices and Radiological Health (click "Medical Devices" or "Radiation-Emitting Products" on the homepage).

If you choose to search the entire FDA site, start by clicking "search" on the homepage. If you want basic information, click on "Advanced Search," then limit the search to the "FDA Consumer Magazine" and "FDA Backgrounders." These are general-information articles written to be understood by consumers. For more detailed information, do a general search without specifying parameters. You'll likely get a lot—perhaps hundreds—of page hits, but you can sort through them based on the three-line summary provided for each page. Also, hits are displayed in descending order of relevance, so if you don't find what you are looking for in the first twenty or so documents, chances are the later documents won't help either. (The relevance score is listed below the document summary for each hit—100% is the highest rating.) This general search will give you very specific drug and device information, including reviews, transcripts of meetings in which scientists describe their research findings, and committee reports, as well as consumer information.

To find information about prescription and nonprescription drugs, go to the "Drugs" section of the FDA, which takes you to the homepage for the Center for Drug Evaluation and Research

(CDER). Click the button for "Specific Audiences" first to see what information has been written specifically for consumers. There is, for example, a Consumer Drug Information page that contains basic information about pharmaceutical drugs approved since January 1998. For more detailed information, you'll have to go to the regular Drug Information page, which can be accessed from the CDER starting page, or from the Consumer Drug Information page. Combined, these pages are the best place to find accurate information on what the drug is used for, what side effects might occur, who shouldn't take the drug, and general precautions.

If you go to the "Food" section of the FDA, you'll find information on food safety, food labeling, additives, and dietary supplements. Although this information is of general importance, it doesn't necessarily address specific issues critical for disease treatment. However, people with compromised immune systems may want to review the food safety information to avoid potentially serious food-borne illnesses. (You can also call a toll-free food safety line at 1-888-SAFEFOOD.) From the "Food" starting page, click on the "Consumer Advice" link to find the articles written especially for consumers. If you need more detailed information, click on any of the special program areas listed on the starting page.

To find information about medical devices go directly to the consumer section of the FDA's Medical Devices/Radiological Health section at http://www.fda.gov/cdrh/consumer/index. html. From here, you can search for the device alphabetically. Not many devices are described on this site, but if the one you want is here, the information is accurate and complete. The main part of the Medical Devices/Radiological Health section can be accessed by clicking on the link on the FDA homepage. For consumers, a general search is often worthless, since most of the documents are intended for manufacturers and approval processes. But if you need very specific information on a particular device, look at the corresponding guidance document, which can be located by clicking on "Guidance Documents" under the "Popular Items" pull-down bar, and then doing a search. The Medical Devices/Radiological Health site also contains information about mammography centers, breast implants, and medical device recalls. Look for these areas under the "Special Interest" pull-down bar.

▶ ACTION PLAN—KEEP HANDY THE BEST PHONE NUMBERS AND WEBSITES

1. Take advantage of highly accurate and consumer-friendly government health information by visiting the websites and calling the telephone help lines as often as you need to. Put helpful clearinghouse telephone numbers in a convenient spot, such as your address book or taped to your refrigerator.
2. These sites can be confusing to search. Don't waste time on any one site if you get bogged down in irrelevant or difficult searches; go to one of the government search functions described in chapter 8.
3. When looking for information about medications, check the FDA Human Drugs site first. This is the most accurate information you'll find.
4. If you find a government site that is particularly helpful, bookmark it so you can easily find it again later.
5. Although government information is excellent, it may not always be complete. Use this as one of your starting points for basic information, and move on from there.

8. Internet

Value as a health information source: ★ ★ ★ ★

Effort required: ★ ★ ★ ☆

Accessibility: ★ ★ ★ ★

Good for: Finding any type of health information, including consumer articles, support groups, journal articles, professional and government postings. Always requires vigilance to judge the quality of the information and the reliability of the site.

IT'S difficult to describe the Internet without sounding like the start of a bad joke. The Internet is so big . . . (How big is it?) . . . that it has been compared to the ocean—huge, vast, deep, never-ending, always churning. It contains whole books, library listings, articles, videos, meeting minutes, reports, brochures, summaries, hospital guidelines, chat rooms, newspapers, advertisements, and more. Just about any type of information you can think of can be found on the Internet, and more is being posted every minute.

The Internet is so important . . . (How important is it?) . . . that its impact has been likened to the development of the telephone or television—connecting people through e-mail and providing mass communication on a grand scale. Why wait for the evening news or the morning paper to hear what's going on in the world? The same news reports used by television and newspaper writers are posted throughout the day on the Internet.

The Internet is so influential . . . (How influential is it?) . . . that some physicians believe it alone is responsible for the shift from doctor-centered paternalism to doctor-patient partnerships. With the Internet, patients have immediate access to virtually all health information that is available, from anywhere in the world. And with that knowledge comes power: power to make intelligent treatment decisions, power to challenge questionable medical procedures, and power to seek the best of complementary medicine.

When it comes to health information, the Internet may be the most exciting and useful development since the printing press. And the beauty of it is that anyone can learn to navigate the Net. No one is "too old" to learn new technology. In 1999, scientists at Duke University Medical Center reported that they introduced the Internet in a retirement community with great success. Although these older adults needed more time and assistance getting started, they were able to learn to use the Internet to find information and send and receive e-mail.

"I really think that the future of searching for [health] information is going to be on the Web, because it's available to you in the middle of the night," says Susan Love, M.D., author of *Dr. Susan Love's Breast Book*, and director of the Susan Love Breast Cancer Foundation and founder of SusanLoveMD.com, a website for women. "You can search right away."

Once you become proficient at navigating the Internet, you'll discover a sense of freedom similar to when you first got your driver's license. Yes, you'll go slow for a while and wonder how you'll ever gain total control over the thing. But with enough practice, you'll be racing around like a pro. The rest of this chapter will guide you past the pitfalls of the Internet (yes, unfortunately, there are some) and tell you the best ways to find the most valuable health information. (Many wonderful books have been written about how to hook up a computer, the mechanics of the Internet, how to find a good Internet service provider [ISP], and the other nuts and bolts of computers and the World Wide Web. If you have questions in any of these areas, browse the computer section of your local bookshop or library for books that answer your concerns. In the near future, there will be a variety of easy-to-use Internet devices that will be a breeze to hook up. You won't even need a computer to use the Internet.)

Quality, Ethics, and Privacy on the Internet

As wonderful as the Internet is, there are some safety concerns you need to be aware of. Despite media attention paid to computer viruses and Internet stalkers, the average person is not usually affected by these threats. Yes, they are out there, but if you don't download software off the Internet or open attachments on suspicious e-mail, there's virtually no way a virus can get into your computer. And you can avoid dangerous people on the Internet the same way you do on the street—by not talking to strangers and not giving out any personal information.

The greatest danger of the Internet is information that is biased, misleading, wrong, dangerous, or downright life-threatening. Of course, dangerous information is harmful only if you believe it and use it in ways that are not in your best interests.

"There is more unreliable and erroneous information on the Internet on almost all health-related issues than there is good information," says Neil B. Mehta, M.D., a physician in the Department of General Internal Medicine at the Cleveland Clinic Foundation. "There may be very Web-savvy or health-savvy patients who are able to differentiate [the good from the bad information], but I think it's probably true that, for most people, it's very difficult. The Internet is considered high tech. Oftentimes, if you read something in the newspaper, you may not believe it. But because the Internet is associated with computers, people may take the same information and believe it a little bit more."

Every physician interviewed expressed similar concerns about health information on the Internet. The goal should not be to avoid the Internet but to learn how to differentiate high-quality, reliable information from misleading or potentially harmful information—or as Mary Jo Deering, Ph.D., director of health communication and telehealth in the Department of Health and Human Services likes to put it, to be able to tell the difference between "the good, the bad, and the ugly."

In general, "good" information is based on solid scientific research. When presented on the Internet, good information is written or endorsed by a reputable person, agency, or organization with no financial or political bias. Standard good sources of health information are the U.S. government, medical specialty societies like the American Cancer Society, universities, hospitals and medical centers (as long as they are not "selling" their programs), and nonprofit disease organizations. All commercial and personal health information sites need to be carefully evaluated for quality, reliability, and timeliness, as described in the guidelines below.

"Bad" information comes from unqualified sources, has little or no scientific backing, and may be tainted by bias or commercial interests. It can be interesting to read, and you may actually learn something from it, but it should not be used as a decision-making aid. For example, if your sister's neighbor tells you that she heard that getting a flu shot was dangerous, that might spur you to do a little extra research about the topic, but it certainly shouldn't influence your flu shot decision. Unless that neighbor is a world-renowned immunity researcher, she is an unqualified source.

Hearsay and health rumors can be spread anywhere, not just on the Internet. Clerks at health food stores and other obviously non-medical people routinely give bad health information because they have minimal—if any—training. Purveyors of "bad" information aren't necessarily bad people. They want to help and are often sincere in their beliefs, but all the sincerity in the world won't make bad information good. Unless a drug, herb, procedure, or other treatment has been subjected to the rigors of scientific study, any benefit from its use can only be said to be anecdote or rumor.

Bad information can also come from individuals or companies with a financial or political ulterior motive. Companies such as pharmaceutical and vitamin manufacturers develop brochures and websites that provide health information, but there is always the question of how much the financial motives of the company influenced the copy. Can you trust that a company that makes a migraine medication will give totally unbiased information about the treatment of migraines? Not really. There is always the possibility of conflict of interest. "A lot of the information that patients get is really promotional material . . . thinly disguised," says Sherrie Kaplan, M.D., associate professor of medicine at Tufts University School of Medicine. It's OK to read the information and learn what you can, but it's a good idea to find an independent source before making a medical decision based on that tainted information.

"Ugly" information is blatantly misleading and potentially harmful. It can come from sincere individuals who inadvertently promote harmful information, or from crass marketers who are looking to make money by duping people who are seriously ill and desperate for a cure. Yes, such people do exist.

"We have always had charlatans. We have always had frauds. But now, with the Internet, we have the possibility of having these charlatans, con artists, come right into the home of the desperate and unsuspecting patient," says Maurie Markman, M.D., director of the Cleveland Clinic Taussig Cancer Center. "What they say they offer is hope, cures, miraculous this-and-that, but many of these people are just out there trying to sell a product."

These charlatans can put up a fancy website that looks as authentic and authoritative as any other—sometimes more so. "Some of these [websites] are really impressive," says Dr. Markman. "Multicolors, multimedia, movies, sound bites—all the things that you could think of to get people impressed with the technology that have nothing whatsoever to do with the quality of the content. And the public would have no way of knowing."

A good way to recognize "ugly" information in any of its forms is if it claims to have found a cure for a disease (especially if the cure is said to be "secret," or unknown, or suppressed by doctors). Also, ugly information often encourages people not to tell their doctors about the treatment, or advises patients to stop seeing their traditional doctor in favor of this new, supposedly progressive treatment. Don't buy into it, no matter how good it sounds. If you feel persuaded by a sales pitch, remember that your goal is to stay in a partnership with your doctor. Talk with him or her about what you read before trying new options.

Website Evaluation Guidelines

The difficulty of judging which sites are "good," "bad," or "ugly" has not escaped the notice of government and commercial organizations. In response, various groups—including the Internet Healthcare Coalition, Health on the Net Foundation, and Hi-Ethics (Health Internet Ethics)—are developing guidelines for ethical standards. The idea is that once the guidelines are presented, all reputable health information providers will sign on to uphold a definitive set of principles that will guide content, advertising, commerce, and privacy practices.

Unfortunately, ethics are currently rather lax on the Internet, which means that the consumer needs to be extra vigilant when judging how trustworthy websites are. Most experts are recommending cautiousness and suggest that patients look at each website with a highly critical eye.

Certain types of websites are more reliable than others:

• *U.S. government health information sites* provide high-quality, reliable, and trustworthy information. Some articles may be outdated, but this can be checked by looking for the "last updated" date. See chapter 7 for more information about government sources. (If the website address ends in .gov [versus .com], you can trust that it is a government site.)

• *Medical specialty societies*—such as the American Medical Association (and its associated website, www.medem.com), the American College of Family Physicians, and the American Academy of Dermatology—also consistently provide high-quality, reliable, and trustworthy health information. No need to be concerned with quality issues. (Society web addresses usually end in .org.)

• *Sites run by well-known nonprofit disease organizations* (such as the American Cancer Society, American Diabetes Association, American Heart Association) are usually highly reliable and trustworthy. There is no need to be concerned about quality of information. Watch out for for-profit organizations whose names are similar to that of the nonprofits. See chapter 10 for more information about associations and organizations. (Many websites that end in .org [versus .com] are not-for-profit organizations, although that has been changing in the past few years. You can no longer trust that a .org website doesn't have commercial interests.)

• *University and medical school websites* are also reliable and trustworthy. Although the information is good, there is the possibility that only a single point of view may be expressed, depending on a particular scientist's or department's biases. For example, a medical school's surgical oncology website may discuss only surgical options for treating cancer and give very little information about chemotherapy or radiation. The surgical information will be valuable, but you may need to find the missing information from other sources. (All university and medical website addresses end in .edu.)

• *Hospital and medical center websites* are generally highly reliable and trustworthy, but you should watch for blatant selling of particular programs and services. As with university and medical school sites, watch for single-point-of-view biases. (Hospital and medical center web addresses usually end in either .org or .edu [if it is closely affiliated with a medical school].)

• *Consumer health information websites* need to be closely examined on a number of different points. The quality, reliability, and trustworthiness can vary quite a bit from one to another. The larger sites—such as InteliHealth, Mayo Clinic, and WebMD—provide information written especially for a consumer audience that is usually accurate. Sites that have formal partnerships with respected major educational or health institutions tend to be a little more trustworthy because the information is often reviewed by experts from those institutions. But even the best sites may have problems related to privacy and conflict of interest. Some sites have been investigated for allowing advertisers to track your movements on the Web. This is particularly true of those that require you to register with your name, address, and e-mail. A report by the California HealthCare Foundation released in February 2000 found that many websites don't have privacy policies, and the ones that do don't necessarily enforce them. Conflict-of-interest problems can also arise. You'll notice that some sites are filled with advertisements, and it may be difficult to tell what is valuable information and what is simply a sales pitch. The concern is heightened if the same company that owns the website owns or is in a financial partnership with other related businesses. For example, if a company that owns a health website also owns a company that sells vitamin supplements, is the site more likely to post articles that promote vitamins? Maybe, maybe not. That's why it is important to look for signs of how trustworthy the site is (see guidelines below). There promises to be a shake-up and consolidation soon in the area of commercial health information websites for consumers. As of this writing, companies are scrambling to survive. Some of the currently popular sites will disappear entirely, others will develop new partnerships and offer different products for sale, and still others will attempt to change their revenue model entirely to stay afloat amid competition. (Large commercial health website addresses usually end in .com, but some may end in .org.)

• *Sites run by companies that create and/or sell health-related products* must always be closely scrutinized. These can include companies that manufacture or sell pharmaceuticals, vitamin/mineral supplements, herbs, medical devices, or health aids. Very few of these product sites provide valuable information that can't be found elsewhere. The typical product site is little more than a public relations strategy, with weak articles, few links to more reliable sources, and plenty of product marketing. As a general rule, avoid these sites as a source of health information. (Product sites are supposed to end in .com—although, lately, some are arranging for .org endings. The rules are becoming lax.)

• *Consumer-run health or disease-specific sites* are a total mixed bag. Some are carefully written, screened by a physician, and have the backing of larger organizations. Others are little more than outlets for disgruntled patients to rant. Unless a site is explicitly recommended by a physician or one of the highly reliable websites, it's best to avoid it. Patients who go through the trouble of setting up a website are usually passionate about their cause, and that passion can easily result in a lack of perspective when it comes to dispensing medical information. Use the guidelines below to guide your evaluation. These sites often have a section for patient stories where other people get to tell what affect the disease has had on their lives. Unfortunately, people who have had only minor difficulties or an optimistic outcome are less likely to write their stories than people who are in distress. This means that the stories are often more pessimistic, depressing, and discouraging than you would find in the general population. Some can be downright horrifying. Imagine a website that was meant to give information about toasters but only posted stories about toasters that shorted out and caused a kitchen fire. After reading enough stories, you're bound to believe that all toasters are dangerous and ought to be outlawed. Read these sites with a level head, and avoid being sucked in by the passion. If you have concerns about anything you read, talk with your doctor. (These sites also usually end with .com.)

Evaluation Guidelines Checklist

For sites that require further evaluation, there are several signs of quality to look for. You don't need to have all the points checked off, but if fewer than half are present, move on to another site. (*Note:* Don't rely on website ratings you may find on the Internet. The criteria used may not be in your best interest. For example, one group downgraded the rankings of health information companies that did not offer health products for sale on their site. Product sales are hardly the mark of a good website.) Look for:

☐ **Credibility.** Look to see what company or organization is running the website, then judge what biases may be present. As outlined above, U.S. government sources are the most reliable and trustworthy, commercial health information sites are less so, and commercial product sites and sites run by individuals are the least credible.

☐ **Medical advisory boards.** There should be a listing somewhere on the site of physicians who are active in making certain that all the information posted is accurate. Look for these listings under "advisers," "board members," "medical staff," or other similar headings. Check the affiliations of the members—the more prestigious the affiliation, the greater the likelihood that the website is well-respected. Although *having* a medical adviser doesn't always mean that the company *uses* the medical adviser, a very negligent website will most likely lose adviser support in time. Look for statements that describe how the review process takes place. Although these statements are currently rare, they are likely to become common in the future as accuracy concerns are recognized as important.

☐ **Special seals of approval.** You will see sites that brag that they passed the Health on the Net Foundation code (the "HON code") of ethical conduct. To receive this citation, the site must adhere to certain ethical standards, including providing contact addresses, privacy and advertisement statements, and clear information. Although the HON code is a good place to start, there's no guarantee that its policies are actually followed. Consider it the base level of a "good" website. As other codes of conduct and Internet content legislation are established, there will doubtless be other seals of approval for good sites. Each time a website is evaluated and rated worthy of a seal of approval, that provides an extra layer of confidence that the information on the site can be trusted.

☐ **Frequent information updates.** Look for notes about when the information was last updated. Be suspicious of medical information that has not been updated in the past six months.

☐ **Attribution.** Information should be backed up by appropriate sources. Articles should state the names and affiliations of any physicians or scientists interviewed, provide the journal names and publication dates of research studies cited, and/or provide a reference list of sources used in the creation of the article. If you don't know where the information came from, there's no way to know how trustworthy it is.

☐ **Privacy statement.** Read the website's privacy statement and make sure you understand it. The link to it should be prominently displayed on the homepage of the site you are visiting. If there is no privacy statement, or if it's too confusing to understand, skip that site. All reputable sites should want to protect your privacy. The ideal policy statement should include assurances that the company will not collect information about you that can identify you as an individual, will not sell or share your personal information to advertisers or other third parties, and will provide adequate security precautions to protect consumer information from hackers. Privacy is a high-priority item on the development agendas of health care organizations, government, and health information companies, so guidelines and policing efforts will undoubtedly arise in the next few years. Right now, if you have a strong desire to protect your privacy, only visit websites that have strict privacy guidelines and do not require you to submit your name and/or address or "register" for site access.

If you are highly concerned with privacy, modify your browser so that your computer does not automatically accept "cookies." (Consult your browser's information homepage to find out how to turn off the cookie option. It's different for each browser.) Cookies are tiny tracking files that are placed on your home computer when you visit a website. Some are valid only for the length of your stay on that website, others stay active for months. The cookie acts almost like an electronic homing device, so the company that placed the cookie can track your movements on the Internet. In most cases, the data is anonymous, and the people doing the tracking only learn where you go, not who you are, so they can't tie you, personally, to the information or the sites where you've been. This information is used to help web advertisers place ads for the kinds of products you are most likely to use on the pages you visit. Many people don't care that a computer somewhere knows the last ten sites they visited. But others care deeply and worry about how the information might be used. By turning off the automatic acceptance of cookies, no tracking information can be placed on your computer. The downside to this is that some websites require you to accept a cookie to go into certain areas, and cookies are often used to make navigation quicker and more personalized. It's your choice.

☐ **Clearly marked and moderate advertising.** All website advertising should be immediately recognizable as an advertisement, the same way you can tell that a commercial is different from a television show. (Websites that are designed to be strictly sales tools are the equivalent of television "infomercials." These can be deceptive, and should not be trusted.) Some website homepages seem to have more banner ads (those boxed advertisements that look like bumper stickers) than medical information. Be wary of these sites—the companies may be more concerned with their advertisers' needs than the needs of the health consumer.

☐ **Clearly stated protection from bias policy.** Somewhere in the website's policy information should be a statement concerning how editorial content (the medical information included on the site) is kept separate from any advertising or partnership considerations. There's no guarantee that the policy is strictly followed, but including it is a good-faith effort that the bias issue has been addressed within the company. Further, any political or financial partnerships should be disclosed, including related corporations, lobbying groups, or other special interest groups.

☐ **Easy to understand and use.** If you don't understand the layout of the website, if the links are hard to follow, or if the information is not written clearly, skip the site. There are many well-designed sites that can offer the same information. Don't waste your time trying to navigate through an electronic swamp.

☐ **Contact information.** There should be some way for you to get in touch with the website managers in case of questions. Look for the "Contact us" or similar page.

During your website evaluation process, don't be impressed by sites that contain lots of links to other sites. Any website can link to another, and no link should be construed as an endorsement by the linked website. (For example, if a website links to the American Cancer Society, that doesn't mean that the American Cancer Society necessarily approves of that website.)

Another highly important piece of advice is that you should never go to the Web for a diagnosis. Any online doctor or other health professional who claims to be able to diagnose a disease without examining you in person is practicing bad medicine. Steer away from these sites.

Look for consensus among the sites you visit. Good health information websites use solid scientific information as their foundation. This type of information should not vary from one site to another. Compare the information you find about your disease from various sites. If they differ enough to make you ask questions, then something is wrong. Always check back with your physician if you find conflicting information.

Many health information sites are starting to offer a service where you can keep your health records online. The format is similar to the Personal Health Log described in chapter 4, except that these logs are kept online at the website. Reactions from physicians and health professionals to these online records have been mixed. Everyone believes it is a good idea to keep a record of some sort, but there are major privacy issues involved. Right now, consumers cannot be certain that their online records will not be lost, read by people who work for the website, or hacked by outsiders. And what happens to your records if the website that contains your health record goes bankrupt or simply shuts down? There may be more privacy and security regulations put into place in the future, but for now it's up to consumers to protect themselves. "Consumers should always press to have a version that resides on their own computer . . . not just rely on someone else's server," says Dr. Mary Jo Deering. The form your record-keeping takes is up to you. If there is a way to download the information onto your computer and keep duplicate records, and if you are comfortable with this intensive interaction with your computer, online record-keeping may be right for you. Otherwise, use the Personal Health Log forms included in this book.

Online Support Groups

Online support groups and bulletin boards have different sets of concerns. Because these sites are often not managed by physicians or other health professionals, there is always the risk that someone may inadvertently give out bad, dangerous, or unduly frightening information. "Also, what can happen is a lot of people masquerade as patients or sufferers and post misinformation related to medications that are supposed to be miraculous cures," says Dr. Neil Mehta. "That is scary. I've seen it happen . . . and since [the information] seems to be coming from a peer, the information is very attractive." Support groups can also be a valuable source of inspiration and information. They tend to work best if they are physician-moderated, or sponsored by a hospital, university, or other well-respected group. Patient-run support groups can be valuable if they primarily provide moral and emotional support. Be very wary of support groups where alternative cures are posted regularly. If you have any questions, talk with your physician. (For more information about support groups, see chapter 14.)

Remember that the Internet is just one information-gathering tool. Don't use Internet information exclusively to make decisions about your medical treatment. And don't add additional treatments you find on the Net, even seemingly harmless herbs or vitamins, without talking it over with your doctor. Some herbs and supplements can have interactions with prescription medications, or can affect the way your body responds to chemotherapy, insulin, or other treatments. (For more information about complementary treatments, see chapter 13.)

How to Search the Internet for Health Information

Every site on the Internet has a specific address or URL (for Uniform Resource Locator), the same way every telephone has a telephone number. With telephone numbers, if you know the number you wish to call, you simply press in the numbers. If you don't know the number, you can check your personal address book, call directory assistance, or look in the telephone book.

The process is similar for URLs. If you know the address of the website you wish to visit, you simply type it into the address bar that's part of your browser. If you don't know the address from memory, you can look it up in your personal online address book (the "Favorites" or "Bookmarked" items), do a search on a search engine (such as Google, Yahoo!, Excite, AltaVista, or Lycos), or search on a health information locator site. It might also help to add a page to your Personal Health Log's journal section where you record the URLs of the sites you most often visit.

Everyone eventually develops his or her own style for searching the Internet, but there are certain guidelines that can make the search more efficient, especially when searching for health information. Use the recommendations here as a starting point, but feel free to modify the search according to your needs.

Ask your doctor what websites he or she might recommend: Doctors often have their own websites, like to refer patients to Web pages associated with their hospital or medical center, or know sites that they have found to be particularly helpful to their patients. Getting the addresses from your doctor can save you time and worry, and can give you an idea of what your doctor considers "good" information about your condition. You can always continue the search from there.

Know your keywords and search options: No matter where you search on the Internet, you need to have a solid idea of exactly what you are looking for. Each searchable site has a blank search bar that requires you to type in keywords to guide the search. In the beginning, when you are looking for basic information, the keywords should be broad and simple. For example, if you are interested in asthma, your main keyword will be "asthma." If you are searching for information on osteoporosis, a disease in which bone density decreases, the initial keywords could be "osteoporosis" and "bone density." Many sites have A-to-Z search functions, and it's often good to start with those so you can browse through lists without coming up with your own keywords.

As you begin to understand your condition better, other keywords will become important. For example, you may start adding certain treatments, physician's names, or medication names to your keyword list. You may learn that rheumatoid arthritis is a form of "autoimmune disorder," so that term can be added to your list. Keep and update your own list of keywords in your Personal Health Log.

The more specific your keywords are, the more focused the information will be, but you'll also get fewer "hits"—the websites or pages that are found in response to your search. And remember that any search function is only as good as the people who program it. You may find that keywords that return dozens of hits on one website may not find any in another not because the information isn't there but because different keywords may be used. For example, "high blood pressure" and "hypertension" are the same condition, but they may turn up different hits from different searches. It's best to keep a flexible attitude when searching the Internet; if one set of keywords doesn't work, try another. If a site turns up only two links, search elsewhere. Even the large search engines differ dramatically in the type and number of hits produced for the same set of keywords.

Once you're past the basic search and need to focus on a specific area, try combining keywords. Advanced search screens will allow you to narrow your search by using "and," "not," and "or" (often in capital letters) to further define what you are searching for. (You may see this referred to as Boolean Logic.) These three little words tell the search program how to search for your keywords by expanding or limiting the choices. For example: There is a group of people in this world who have heart disease. There is also a group of people in this world who have diabetes. Here is a visual representation of what I mean:

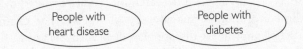

But there is also a group of people who have both heart disease and diabetes. This is often illustrated by having the ovals overlap. The area that is shaded falls within both the heart disease oval *and* the diabetes oval. This represents the group of people who have both disorders. Again, a visual illustration:

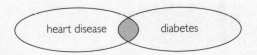

• Use "AND" (in all capital letters) if you want to search for the small group of articles that deal with *both* heart disease and diabetes. Type *"heart disease" AND diabetes* in the search bar. This will return only articles that discuss both diseases. This is helpful when you want to narrow your search. You can, for example, look for information about your condition *and* a particular medication, which would turn up only articles about using that medication to treat your condition.

• Use "OR" (in all capital letters) if you want to search for articles that deal with *either* heart disease or diabetes. Type *"heart disease" OR diabetes* in the search bar. This will return all articles in both groups. This is helpful when you want to expand your search. For example, you can look for high blood pressure (type in "OR") hypertension, and get all articles, regardless of how the websites refer to the condition.

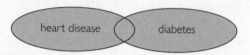

• Use "NOT" if you want to search for articles on heart disease but eliminate another subcategory of disease. For example, many articles on heart disease also deal with diabetes. If you don't have diabetes, but half the articles in your search concern diabetes, you can eliminate those by using "NOT." Type *"heart disease" NOT diabetes* in the search bar. This will return only heart disease articles in which diabetes is not mentioned. This is helpful if you find your search keeps turning up irrelevant information. For another example, *"your condition NOT children"* should weed out articles that deal with a pediatric population.

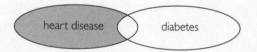

Use search shortcuts: When typing your keywords into a search bar, there are a few common rules that can make your search easier. First, some searches look for *any* of the words you put in the search bar while others look for *all* the words—but not necessarily in the same order you typed them. To look for specific key phrases, type quote marks (" ") around the words. For example, simply typing *rheumatoid arthritis* in some search engines will return articles on rheumatoid arthritis, but also irrelevant articles on other *rheumatoid* diseases and non-rheumatoid *arthritis*. But if you type *"rheumatoid arthritis"* with the quote marks, the search engine will return only articles that contain both words, in that order. Second, it is often possible to use a wild card character to fill in for missing letters. This is most useful if you don't know the exact spelling of the word or if the word has several possible endings you'd like to search. For example, many sites use the asterisk (*) as a wild card character. (Check the "Help" section of the websites you search for the characters they use.) In this case, typing "myelo*" will return hits with the words *myeloma, myeloblast, myeloblastic leukemia, myelocele,* and other similar words. Third, don't bother using the words *a, an,* or *the*. Most computer programs skip these anyway. Finally, be very careful about spelling. Computers can be dumb machines that do only what you tell them to do; they won't know that when you typed "blook" you meant "blood." The program will look for "blook." If you get few or no hits on a search, check your spelling. (Some newer Internet Explorer programs do spelling correction or a nearest-word search, so even bad spelling may not matter in the future.)

Start by searching the most reliable, trustworthy sites first: As mentioned earlier, sites can vary greatly in the quality of information they provide, but certain sites are consistently reliable. The best place to start searching is with the U.S. government's health information locator, *healthfinder* (www.healthfinder.gov).

This site was developed to take advantage of the new Internet technology by providing a gateway to the best, most accurate, and most reliable health sites. The *healthfinder* site provides topic lists and a simple search function that point consumers to agencies, organizations, and informational articles based on a stringent set of selection criteria. They refer primarily to U.S. government agencies, national not-for-profit and professional organizations that serve the public interest (such as the American Cancer Society), universities, libraries, and a limited number of carefully screened commercial sites.

You won't find everything you need to know about a specific disease or condition from the links on *healthfinder,* but all the referred websites are prescreened for quality and value, so you can be confident that you're starting out on a solid, scientific footing. You will also become comfortable with searching by different strategies, and will become familiar with the most reputable information sources.

The U.S. government also has two other sites that are particularly helpful when starting a search: the MEDLINEplus Health Information site and the National Women's Health Information Center.

MEDLINEplus (http://medlineplus.nlm.nih.gov/medlineplus/) provides information on hundreds of diseases, conditions, and wellness issues as well as links to many helpful resources, including medical dictionaries and encyclopedias, doctor and dentist directories, hospital and organization directories, and medical databases. The information and directories are from high-quality sources, so accuracy and reliability are virtually assured.

The National Women's Health Information Center (www.4women.gov) offers information and resource services on women's health issues, including gynecological disorders, fertility, and eating disorders, as well as disease information. Again, the information is highly accurate, reliable, and trustworthy.

The American Medical Association websites (www.ama-assn. org and www.medem.com) offer consumer health information that has been specially prepared for or by the AMA. All information here can be trusted. In fact, many government sites link to the AMA's website.

Use a standard search engine: Search engines are giant software programs that search the Web for your keywords and match them to titles or words in other websites or documents. Each search engine uses a different program, and so the number and type of documents or sites that will be returned will vary from one to another. They usually allow both simple and advanced searches. Each search engine has a help page that describes how to use it, so click on "Help" if you need it. Some of the currently popular search engines are Google (www.google.com), Yahoo (www.yahoo.com), Excite (www.excite.com), and AltaVista (www.altavista.com). If you go to one of the search engines and do a search for "search engines," you'll find the names of others. (No doubt new search engines will be devised over the next few years, and some of these may disappear, but the principle behind them will remain generally the same.)

Try out several search engines with the same set of keywords to see how well they respond to your needs. This type of comparison will show you which are the easiest to use, which return the most accurate hits, and which give mostly "garbage" or hits that are not useful. Most people find that they tend to use the same two or three search engines exclusively. (There are meta-search engines, such as MetaCrawler or Dogpile, which pull together several individual search engines. These are not recommended. While it may seem that they will help you cover more ground more quickly, they are often difficult to use and may miss some of the sites you need most.)

No matter which search engine you use, chances are you'll get dozens, if not hundreds or thousands, of hits on a broad search. If you get more hits than you're comfortable dealing with, try narrowing your search by adding keywords, or by using the AND, NOT, and OR functions as described above. How each hit is described will also vary by search engine. The description may include the name of the site or page, the URL, a brief description of what the site contains, and/or the name of the sponsoring organization. Often you'll be able to tell what type of site it is (government, university, nonprofit organization) from the description or URL. If not enough information is given but the site seems interesting, click the link to go directly to the site. Once there, you can use the guidelines above to evaluate how reliable and trustworthy the information is likely to be. To return to the previous page, simply click the "Back" button on your browser.

Follow links to other high-quality sites: Every site offers links to other similar sites. These are the Web addresses that, if you click on them, will take you to that site. Links can be pictures, icons, or words that are highlighted or underlined. This is a great way to discover other good sites. The best websites—government sites, medical specialty societies, medical schools, and universities—will not usually link to bad sites, so their links can be trusted. But the farther down the reliability scale you go, the less trustworthy the linked sites may be. Since there are no rules about which sites can link up with other sites, some bad sites may actually link to good sites, but they can also link to other bad sites. If the link is dubious, simply do your own evaluation of the site once you get there.

Once you find a particularly helpful site, you can print the pages you want to keep, and then "bookmark" the site using the "Bookmark" or "Favorites" option on your browser. This will place the URL of your most useful sites in a special file on the computer so you can return to those sites with just the click of a mouse key. If you prefer, you can also write your favorite Web addresses in your Personal Health Log.

You can also keep track of complicated searches in your PHL. For example, if you have found that certain websites have turned out to be dead-ends, note that in your PHL so you don't have to repeat that frustrating process in the future.

Many people are nervous about being on the Internet. They are afraid that they will somehow get trapped on a site, or get lost, or do something to ruin the program. Don't worry. You really can't make any mistakes on the Internet. Wherever you go on the Web, you can always get back to where you were by clicking on the "Back" button of your browser (several times if necessary), or by retyping the original URL in the address bar of your browser.

There is a tremendous amount of information on the Internet, and you'll find that different types of information and websites will be valuable to you at different times. Information that is too complex for you to understand today may seem simple two months from now, after you've had more experience reading medical terminology; and articles that you printed and saved three weeks ago may seem worthless once you understand the specifics of your condition better.

Try to pace yourself when gathering information. Unless you are facing a life-threatening disease, one that requires that you gather as much information as you can immediately, go slowly, stick with the best websites, find information that matches your comfort level, then go back periodically to find the next level of information. At some point you'll undoubtedly find yourself either frustrated or overwhelmed by the process. That is entirely normal. Just remember, you can always turn off the computer and come back another day. If you feel that you have the time and are running into stumbling blocks on the Internet, you may want to take a beginning computing class at your local community center or college. There are also many books available that simply list useful medical-site addresses. This may take some confusion out of your search, but beware that these books might not be entirely accurate or up-to-date.

▶ ACTION PLAN—USE YOUR DISCRETION

1. Look carefully at the websites you visit. Evaluate the sites for trustworthiness. Some sources are almost always dependable, such as U.S. government health sites, universities and medical schools, medical specialty societies, and nonprofit disease organizations. All commercial sites should be evaluated using the Internet guidelines.
2. Be especially wary of sites that are strictly designed to sell a product, and avoid sites that claim to have a "secret remedy" or "miracle cure."
3. Guard your privacy on the web. Think twice about visiting sites that require you to "register" by giving your name and other private information before being able to access information. If it does seem valuable, find and read the site's privacy policy and be sure you are comfortable with their use of your personal information.
4. Do not make medical decisions based solely on informa-

tion you find on the Internet. Always discuss your findings
and concerns with your physician.

5. Save the best websites on your computer with the "Favorites" or "Bookmark" option on your browser so you can
   find them easily at a later date. Alternately, write down the
   addresses in your Personal Health Log.

6. Be flexible when searching. Try different keywords if your
   original search turns up few hits.

7. The Internet is a tool. Use it as much or as little as you
   need. You don't have to read everything on the Web.

8. If you become frightened or confused by anything you
   read on the Internet, talk with your doctor.

E-MAIL FOR HEALTH

*E-mail can be a wonderful tool for gathering health information by
allowing you to talk with health experts around the world. Many physicians are hooked into an e-mail system and enjoy e-mail communication because it is so quick and easy to use. Doctors can answer e-mail
anytime they have a free moment, which may be three minutes after
lunch, or at 4:00 in the morning.*

Patients can use e-mail to contact their own doctors to ask
questions or make status reports. They can also e-mail experts in
other states or countries to ask for advice. Many doctors will post
their e-mail addresses on their websites to encourage this type of
communication. And because they can take as long as they want to
compose an e-mail message, many patients feel more comfortable
writing than talking on the telephone.

But there are some unspoken rules of e-mail communication
with physicians you should keep in mind:

- *Don't use e-mail in an emergency.* Your doctor may read e-mail
  only once a week. Call the office or 911 in a true emergency.

- *Don't expect an answer immediately.* Even if the doctor reads
  your message right away, he or she may need time to look at
  your files or research the information you need. This may take

hours or days. If you haven't heard from your doctor after a week and you need a response, call the office.

- *Talk with your doctor about when e-mail is appropriate.* Some doctors don't like e-mail, while others find it a valuable tool for communicating with their patients. Ask your doctor how he or she feels about communicating this way, and when it is appropriate.
- *Be brief.* No physician will have time to read a long, rambling document. Get to the point, give all relevant information, then sign off. A good e-mail can be as short as three sentences. Try to include:

  1. Why you are writing—to ask a question, to report symptoms, to get a referral.
  2. What prompted you to write—physician requested it, saw the physician's name on an Internet site, confused about something you read.
  3. Get to business—ask the question, report the symptom, ask for the referral.
  4. Include relevant information—if asking for a referral, tell the doctor the basics of your condition and where you live. If asking a question, make sure you include any information the doctor might need to answer it. Use short sentences or bullet points if that makes the information easier to read.
  5. What you want the doctor to do—note the symptom in your file, call, or write back with information.
  6. Sign off and give your contact information, including e-mail and telephone number. If the doctor feels the need, he or she may call instead of e-mailing back.

- *Don't write too often.* The doctor is not your pen-pal, and likely has hundreds of patients to deal with. Write only when necessary or when previously agreed upon.
- *Be courteous.* Don't use e-mail to vent your frustrations, pain, or anger. Those emotions are best dealt with in person. If you're angry because you believe you've received poor treatment by the physician, find a new doctor. Don't bad-mouth your old doctor to a new or prospective doctor.

- *Use experts for referrals.* The best cardiac surgeon in the world usually knows the name of the second-best and third-best surgeons. If, during your Internet search, you discover a doctor who seems to be tops in his or her field but you cannot get treatment from that doctor, you can use e-mail to ask for a referral to a top surgeon in your area. Most are happy to give you the names of well-qualified physicians. Do not write to experts and ask for specific advice about your condition, or to complain about your treatment or symptoms, or to ask for a diagnosis. These physicians are busy treating their own patients, and no doctor can make a diagnosis or recommendation without examining you in person.

USING THE INTERNET (MR. HENIG'S INTREPID SEARCH)

At age seventy, Richard Henig is more Internet-savvy than most people I know. In fact, I found Mr. Henig through the Internet. He had posted the story of his search for information and subsequent surgery on a university-sponsored support site for people with aneurysms (State University of West Georgia, http://www.westga.edu/~wmaples/aneurysm.html). When I e-mailed him to ask if he would be interested in being interviewed, he responded within hours, and we discussed how he uses the Internet.

In Mr. Henig's words: Take it from me, the Internet can save your life.

I found out I had an abdominal aortic aneurysm (AAA) when I was sixty-five years old. I had gone to a urologist to check on some kidney stones, and he told me about the AAA. At that point, I had no real knowledge of what it was, but I found out that it was a bulge in the large aortic artery in my abdomen. The vascular surgeon my doctor sent me to said that it was a fairly good-sized one, 3.4 centimeters, and was the type that was likely to rupture, and I would be dead within ten minutes. He told me to come back in three months for a checkup.

I immediately called my family doctor, who told me that the vascular surgeon was exaggerating, and that I should come back in three months for a checkup. Which I did. But during those three months, I got onto the Internet because that first doctor really shook me up, and I decided to start looking to see what I could find.

I went to Yahoo!, which at that time was the main search engine, put in "abdominal aortic aneurysm," and it directed me to a site for a doctor from Columbia University in New York that had a great deal of information, including some questions to ask my doctor. The website also gave me the feeling that all was not lost. I went back to the original doctor, the one who told me I was going to die, to talk some more. I asked him how many AAAs he had treated. His response to me was, "I just saved the life of a ninety-five-year-old woman." I said, "Doctor, that isn't what I asked you. I asked how many AAAs have you done." He said, "I have told you, and that's all I'm going to say about it." At that point, I told this guy he better not bill Medicare, and I walked out of his office.

I immediately went to my family doctor's office, but he was on vacation. At that point I panicked, so I went home, got on the Internet, went again to the Columbia University AAA site, and e-mailed the doctor in charge. I explained to him what I had been told, and that I thought I needed another opinion. He wrote back and said, yes, I did need a second opinion, and he gave me the names of three surgeons he recommended in my area, including one who was a personal friend of his. I chose the one who was the friend.

On my first visit, the surgeon confirmed my aneurysm and its size. I asked him what my chances were. He told me that AAA surgery was the second most common surgery that his department performed, and he had only a 2 percent mortality rate. He told me the chances of a rupture were not significant in AAAs under 5 centimeters, and that I should stop worrying about it. What a difference from the first doctor!

Over a couple of years, I went back to see him, and the aneurysm continued to grow. At that point, I was feeling very comfortable with this surgeon. I'd done a lot more research, and discovered that there was more than one way to treat AAAs, including a less invasive method. I found out everything on the Internet. There were many helpful sites—the Mayo Clinic, the NIH, the Columbia University AAA site, the FDA, and many others. I got my medical education quickly. I figured there's only one person who's going to take care of my health, and that's me, so I damned well better do it right.

I decided which procedure I wanted by carefully following all the information on the Net in regard to the different treatments, including the stories of some folks on a support page who had had the less invasive surgery. But statistics said there was about a 10 to 15 percent failure rate within six months to one year after surgery, which meant that these people had no choice but to go back and have the complete invasive surgery. So I pretty well had made my mind up based on that to have the full invasive surgery right away.

My surgery went well, and I just had my one year checkup. I know that getting on the Internet and finding the Columbia University site was the best thing I could do. The first surgeon had me convinced I was going to die . . . the right surgeon saved my life.

Now, I get to help other people, too. I get e-mail from all over the world from my posting on the AAA support site, asking my advice. I never give them an answer, just a direction to follow. When people who contact the site are about to go through surgery, we e-mail them, build them up, tell them to hang in.

Obviously, I think the Internet is absolutely fabulous. There's so much information out there, so much to learn. The information is there; you have to be aggressive, you have to go after it, and you have to find out. You can do a lot of things if you make the decision that you're going to get involved in taking care of yourself.

9. Medical Journals and MEDLINE

Value as a health information source: ★ ★ ★ ★
Effort required: ★ ★ ★ ★
Accessibility: ★ ★ ☆ ☆

Good for: Detailed and specific medical information, as reported in individual studies. Not for the beginner.

MEDICAL journal articles are the Mount Everest of health information—and you're going to need patience, perseverance, and special training before you can hope to tackle them successfully. But if you take it slowly and follow the guidelines, you'll be able to read and understand much of the same information medical specialists use to make treatment decisions.

What makes journals so challenging? First, they're not meant to be read by the Average Joe. They are written by scientists for other scientists, specialists who have had years of medical school or graduate training that taught them how to think, write, and speak their professional jargon. Words that are perfectly clear to them can sound like a foreign language to the rest of us. But over time, and with the help of a good medical dictionary, it is possible to learn enough "medicalese" to be able to translate the scientific findings into information that's meaningful to you.

The second reason journal articles are so challenging is that they never tell the whole story. Journal articles are tiny slivers of information that come from individual research projects. Many people read an article or two, then jump to premature conclusions based on that limited information. They aren't alone in that tendency—newspapers and other media also jump to premature conclusions, sometimes with near-disastrous results. For example, in the late 1990s, a single article published in a prestigious medical journal described a study in which drugs were able to shrink tumors in mice by cutting off the blood supply to the tumors. Many reports in the media interpreted this to mean that a cure for cancer was right around the corner. The story made headlines across the United States, but it was misleading. Although the research was an important step in cancer research, the conclusions in many instances were erroneous, and tens of thousands of cancer patients were misled into believing the hype. Even if that study was the beginning of an end to cancer, many more studies would be needed to confirm the results and then test it for safety and efficacy in humans.

"Patients and families need to know that one article never makes a new technology the standard of care," says William C. Dooley, M.D., Director of the Johns Hopkins Breast Center. "It takes several articles—from several different institutions scattered around the U.S. and the world finding the same thing—for it to become standard. Look for the review documents that give a more global picture, instead of the individual studies that have numbers and percents." To understand your illness and treatment options, you'll need to read many different articles, absorb the study findings, discuss them with your doctor, and then, only then, make decisions.

The third factor that makes reading journals so difficult is that the information in the articles can be downright frightening. Difficult diseases often have difficult answers. Even the success stories can be intimidating. For example, you may read about an experimental new drug that increases life expectancy for someone suffering from a terminal disease from two months to ten months. It's difficult to read that a disease can cause death so quickly, but the bottom line for people with that disease is that this new option may extend their lives. Your goal is to find all possible options, and then work with your doctor to figure out which is the best for you. Whatever you find, you'll have much of the same information the best doctors have, so you'll be better prepared to make the hard decisions.

It's important to note that not everyone needs to search out and read medical journal articles. If your illness is common, relatively benign, and has standard treatments that work well, there's no reason for you to bother with this portion of the search. For example, if you have been diagnosed with a skin fungus, the disease can be irritating and painful, but a simple antifungal agent is usually enough to take care of the problem in a matter of weeks. But if your illness is serious, unusual, or has several different treatment options, medical journals may be the best source of detailed, current information.

A word of caution: Do not attempt to read medical journals until you have exhausted all other sources of information. To get anything out of this search, you need to have a good basic understanding of your illness and a list of questions or treatment options you need to investigate further. If you try to begin your investigation with medical journals or to accelerate your search before you're fully prepared, you'll only end up confused and frustrated.

Anatomy of a Journal Article

If you are not a scientist, a medical journal article is like nothing you've ever seen before. Reading one is different from reading a newspaper or magazine article.

When scientists conduct research studies, they communicate the results with other scientists through journals. Journals act a little like newspapers in that they publish the latest findings, but they also act as archives where individual articles go "on the record" toward building a full body of knowledge in specific areas.

Not all journals are alike. Just as with books, magazines, and Internet sites, journals have different levels of reliability and respectability. The highest standard for scientific journals is the "peer review" journal. This means that the article was reviewed not only by the editorial staff of the journal but also by other scientists familiar with the subject matter. They check to make sure that the article addresses an important question or issue, that the experiment was well-designed and measured what it was intended to measure, that the statistical analyses were performed correctly, and that the conclusions drawn fit the data. If it fails in any of these areas, the article will not be printed.

How can you tell if a journal is peer reviewed? Depending on what information you start with it can be difficult, but there are a few guidelines you can follow. First, if you found the article via a MEDLINE search (which I will explain in full later), then you can be assured that the journal is of high quality. The director of the National Library of Medicine determines which journals it will include in MEDLINE based on scientific policy and quality. Second, look at the actual journal in a medical library. Each journal lists its review policy somewhere in each issue, usually in the final pages, and the words *peer-reviewed* should appear in that policy statement. Third, if a friend hands you a photocopied article and you don't recognize the journal title, you can check MEDLINE to see if that journal is included (which will mean that it is of high scientific quality). Finally, if you have any question at all about the integrity of the journal, ask your doctor. Most doctors know the reputable journals in their area of specialty. Articles in non-peer-reviewed journals should be read with skepticism.

Each article describes a study designed to answer a very specific scientific question. There are three main types of articles:

1. *Reports of a new, single experiment study.* These generally address narrow questions, such as how two specific chemotherapy regimens compare as a cancer treatment, or the effect of hormone replacement therapy on glycemic control and hypertension in women with diabetes. Although all medical advance-

ments start from a single study, no single study is enough to create a standard of treatment. Look for multiple studies that all say the same thing, or look for reviews or meta-analyses.

2. *Reviews.* These articles look at similar experiments that have been published individually and attempt to draw conclusions about what the "medical truth" is. For example, various studies have been done to discover whether vasectomies increased risk of prostate cancer. Some studies found the answer to be "yes," others said "no." Several review articles examined available evidence, including how well the studies were done, and found that vasectomy does *not* increase risk for prostate cancer. Review articles are, for the most part, more reflective of reality than individual studies, since they take into account a wide range of studies all done on the same topic.

3. *Meta-analysis.* These are similar to review articles in that a meta-analysis attempts to integrate the information from several different sources. The difference is that while review articles look at the big picture made up of the smaller individual parts, a meta-analysis takes information from many individual studies, pools the data from the individual studies, then statistically reanalyzes this massive collection of information. Meta-analyses are controversial, since many scientists believe it isn't right to take data that was gathered from different places at different times under different conditions and throw it all together in a big pot—they feel that the data may not be comparable. Others believe that it is a statistically valid way of looking at the big picture. In general, scientists tend to give a meta-analysis more weight than an individual study, but with the caveat that the results may not accurately reflect reality.

No matter which kind of study is being reported, there is a very specific format for writing up the results. Each article will contain these sections:

- *Abstract:* an overall summary of the article that includes as much detail as the authors and journal editors deem appropriate. Some are only one sentence long and very general, while others can take up nearly a page and provide many details. When you use a database to search for medical journal articles about your illness (see below), you will get to read only the abstract. Usually you can get a good idea of whether the article will give you the information you're looking for based on the abstract alone.

- *Introduction:* tells the reader the background from which the scientists were working, including why they did the research, what questions they were hoping to answer, and what other research has found in the past.

- *Methods:* where scientists tell absolutely everything they did while conducting the experiment. This will include some information you'll need to know to judge how relevant the study was to your situation. For example, it will tell how many subjects were in the experiment, whether they studied men or women or both, the ages of the people studied, and the dosages of medications given.

- *Results:* the part of the article where the scientists tell what they discovered, using statistics to tell the story. Graphs and charts can also be found in this section.

- *Conclusion/Discussion:* where the scientist tells (in relatively plain language) what his or her statistics mean. There is usually a discussion about what the study contributes to the body of medical knowledge and what future questions need to be answered.

- *References:* lists all previously published articles that were cited in the body of the paper.

One recent trend among some journals is to provide a "Patient Page," an interpretation of selected studies presented in common English for the average person to read. This is good news for health consumers because it signals a willingness on the part of journals to allow patients better access to the research by making it more understandable. Look for these pages on specific journal websites, especially those associated with the American Medical Association (www.ama-assn.org).

How to Read a Journal Article

Each section of a journal article plays an important role in telling scientists why the research was done, how it was done, and what it showed. As you become more familiar with medical journal articles, you'll find that deciphering what they mean becomes easier. If you are comfortable reading the article all the way through, from start to finish, please do. You'll find a wealth of knowledge in each section. But if you are like many people looking for a simple way to understand complex health information, you'll want to use the "shortcuts":

• *Read the title.* In any search, you'll first be presented with a large number of article titles. Your first cut comes at this very basic level. If you don't understand the title with the help of a medical dictionary, you won't understand the article, so skip that one. That doesn't mean it isn't valuable on some scientific level, but an article won't do you any good unless you can understand what it is saying. When you get more experience with medical information you may want to do another search and try these articles again, but for now, move on. Sometimes a search turns up odd or totally irrelevant titles, and those will be easy to weed out. From the ones that appear to be related to your interests, pull up the abstract.

• *Look at the list of authors and their affiliations.* After a while, you may find that certain authors keep popping up. Keep track of these names—those doctors are probably among the best in their field. The same thing is true of the affiliations (where the scientists are from). If you find that many of the articles you're interested in were written by scientists from the same one or two institutions (such as Memorial Sloan-Kettering or the Mayo Clinic), then chances are those institutions are centers of excellence for your disease. These may be places you'll want to visit in the future for treatment or second opinions (see chapter 12).

• *Read the abstract all the way through.* Since it is generally very short, this won't take much time, and it will usually give you an even better indication of whether the article is appropriate for you. It may not be. You may find that an article that sounded good from its title actually was a study of mice, or looked at a different form of your disease. That will become clear from reading the abstract. You will also usually learn the results of the study, positive or negative (although most studies publish only positive results, unless they are debunking a commonly held belief). If, after reading the abstract, you feel that the article is exactly what you are looking for, print it to keep for future reference, and then put the electronic version on the MEDLINE "clipboard" (see below for more instructions on using MEDLINE). Of all the abstracts you save, narrow your choices down to the five to ten articles that seem to deal most closely with your problem, and then find the full-text articles. In a perfect world, all the information you need would be contained in the abstract alone. Many times it will be, but you can't count on it. One study that looked at the accuracy of abstracts found that a significant proportion of them—18 to 68 percent—had inconsistencies or listed information not stated in the article. You can find articles in a medical or consumer health library (see chapter 5) or order them from Loansome Doc (see "Miscellaneous Tips" below). In a few cases, the full text of a journal is offered online. The U.S. government has set up an Internet site called PubMed Central, which acts as a centralized place to find full-text online medical journals, free of charge. Several journals are already available there, and many more will likely sign up as online publishing and information searching become the norm. Check this site—http://www.pubmedcentral.nih.gov—to see if the journal you are looking for is available free before paying for articles or making a special trip to the library.

• *Read the introduction* once you have the full article in front of you. This will explain why the article is important and define the question the research sought to answer. If the study no longer sounds as though it pertains to you, dump it and move on to the next one. Take your time reading this section. Note the previous studies that are cited here—you may want to go

back and read these studies as well. They are listed at the back
of the paper in the Reference section.

• *Skip the methodology and results sections for now.*

• *Read the conclusion or discussion section entirely* (it immediately follows the Results section). This section should give you
a good idea of what the results of the study were and what the
researchers think they mean in terms of the bigger scientific
picture.

• *Crystallize your thinking or clarify your understanding* by
writing a couple of sentences describing what the overall outcome of the study was; pay close attention to differences in
subjects or treatments offered. For example, if the treatment
that was described in a journal article relieved pain in pre-
menopausal women but not postmenopausal women, make
sure you write that down—it may become important when
making decisions later. If you feel you cannot summarize the
study for yourself, read it again more slowly.

• *For additional information about the study*, go back and read
the Methods and Results sections. These sections are the equivalent of reading the fine print in a contract and have a tremendous amount of detail that most patients won't need. The most
important information in the Methods section is the type of
experimental design used (see "Types of Scientific Studies," page
162), and the number and type of subjects used. The Results
section contains the complete statistical report (see chapter 15).
Most of the time, you'll never have to read these sections, but
they are there if you want them.

When you feel you understand the article, and if it has meaning for you and your condition, copy it, put it in your Personal
Health Log, and move on to the next article. After you have
several articles that seem important to your condition, compare
what they say. Do they all say basically the same thing or do they
contradict one another? Is there a review article that can piece
them all together for you? Try to form a "big picture" view of
the information for yourself by understanding the differences
among the studies, and how each pertains to your condition.

Bring any questions, issues, or articles that are particularly interesting to your physician. Doctors agree that one of their greatest frustrations is when patients walk into their office with fifty different articles that they didn't take the time to read carefully enough to know that they didn't apply. Bring no more than three articles or questions about articles to a visit. If you have more questions than that, ask the doctor what would be the best way to get your questions answered.

How to Find Journal Articles: MEDLINE

The easy way to get appropriate articles is to have a trained medical librarian or for-fee search company do the research and find them for you (see chapters 5 and 10). But if you enjoy the search process, or if you don't have ready access to a consumer health library, or if you are in a hurry, you're going to need to learn how to use the online medical database MEDLINE.

Back before most people had access to the Internet, MEDLINE was a complex database that charged users a pretty steep fee. And not just anyone could turn on a computer and start searching. Specialized classes were held to teach medical librarians the ins and outs of the database and the special codes that were needed to do research. Now, thanks to the National Library of Medicine, anyone can search through a listing of more than 11 million article references, or citations, in MEDLINE and other medical databases *without cost*. And even better, the search functions have been simplified.

MEDLINE can be accessed through any computer with an Internet connection. The service is free and unlimited, and you can print out all the citations you want—as long as they are for your personal use only. (Please read the "Restrictions on Use" disclaimer found at the bottom of the MEDLINE homepage.) If you do not have a computer at home, check your local library. This is one time where a computer or terminal is necessary—medical citations are no longer compiled in hard copy. Take heart: Although the instructions seem long, involved, and difficult, the actual search is very easy. Read through the instructions, then try your own search or follow along with the example search given at the end of this chapter.

To begin searching MEDLINE, go to the Internet site for the National Library of Medicine's "PubMed" search service at http://www.ncbi.nlm.nih.gov/entrez. (This site has been revamped in the past few years, and the National Library of Medicine promises to keep the site updated. If this URL has become outdated, go to http://www.nlm.nih.gov, the homepage for the National Library of Medicine, and look for the link to MEDLINE.)

A basic search on MEDLINE is pretty simple, and that's what will be discussed here. There are other, more involved ways of searching that allow physicians and scientists to find the information they need quickly, but for most patients' needs, the simpler the better. The website has wonderful support options that can help you should you run into any problems, have any questions, or want to explore other search options. The "Help" and "FAQ" (for Frequently Asked Questions) sections on the homepage describe everything you need to know to do a complete MEDLINE search.

The first step to doing a MEDLINE search is to define your question. Remember, MEDLINE is not the place to go to find general information; you should already have a good idea of what your disease is, what the basic treatment options are, and what your remaining questions are. The narrower the question, the better the chances are that you'll find an answer through MEDLINE. You can't, for example, try to answer broad questions such as "What are all the treatment options for rheumatoid arthritis," or "How can I stop diarrhea," or "What are ascites?" In these cases, the search will yield far too many articles, most of which will be useless and only waste your time. These questions are better answered by books, government sources, or your doctor. MEDLINE works best if you can define a very specific question that will help you make a particular medical decision. Some examples of specific questions:

- "What is the maximum tolerated dose of irinotecan combined with 5-FU and leucovorin used to treat colon cancer?" (Keywords: colon cancer, irinotecan, 5-FU, leucovorin, dosage, maximum tolerated.)
- "Is there an alternative to amputation for nonhealing foot wounds resulting from diabetic neuropathy?" (Keywords: diabetes, neuropathy, foot wounds, nonhealing, treatment, amputation.)
- "Are my chances of getting a breast cancer relapse greater if I only have a sentinel node biopsy, compared to axillary node dissection?" (Keywords: breast cancer, biopsy, sentinel node, axillary node dissection.)
- "How successful are pancreas transplants to treat diabetes?" (Keywords: pancreas, transplant, diabetes.)

Each person will have a different set of questions, depending on his or her disease or condition and the particular circumstances of that individual. Work to make your questions as specific as you can.

Research one question at a time to minimize confusion. From your question, create a list of keywords. These are the words that you will plug into the database to try to answer your question. Don't just keep them in your head; write them down on a piece of paper. The first keyword should always be the specific name of your disease, followed by the common name of your disease. For example, "lobular carcinoma" followed by "breast cancer," or "diabetic neuropathy" followed by "nerve damage."

After that, list any and all medical terms or phrases that fit your question. Include exact drug names (both brand and generic), treatment types, and other words critical to defining the search (see keywords in the sample questions listed above). You may not need all these words, or you may need to add more words later, but this gives you a place to start.

On the MEDLINE homepage, there is a "Search" bar across the top of the page that reads:

Search PubMed for [_____] [Go] [Clear]

You always want to search "PubMed," so don't change what's in that box. In the long blank search box, enter your keywords. You should leave a space between each keyword, but do not include any punctuation. Start by typing in the two or three keywords that best define your question. (The program assumes you want to search for all those words, so you do not have to use "AND" between your keywords.) If you make a mistake, either correct it the way you would in a word-processing program, or click on the "Clear" box. When you are ready for MEDLINE to search, click "Go."

MEDLINE will return a list of article titles that fit your keywords. Read through the titles, and pull up the abstracts of any articles that sound promising by clicking on the authors' names. (Some articles won't have abstracts, so the title is all you'll have to go by. These are usually articles that deal with less technical issues or very old articles.) If after reading the abstract the article still sounds interesting, temporarily save it by placing it on the MEDLINE "clipboard."

MEDLINE CLIPBOARD

From the screen where you are reading the abstract, click on the box that says "Add to Clipboard" just above the titles list. You can also add to the clipboard from the page that lists all the titles by first clicking in the small blank box to the left of the authors' names (a check mark will appear in the box) and then clicking on the "Add to Clipboard" box. You must add these to your clipboard before moving on to the next page of titles, otherwise you'll lose them. To see what you have on your clipboard, click on the word *Clipboard* under the long search box at the top of the page. All your clipboard titles will be cleared after an hour of no usage, so make sure you print out or save what you need if you plan to end or delay your search. To save your clipboard information directly to your computer or a disk, go into the clipboard and click on the "Save" button.

If no titles are returned after your initial search, check to make sure you spelled the keywords correctly (you can check this in the box at the top of the page or go back to the PubMed homepage). Correct any mistakes and try again. If your spelling was correct, try broadening your search by reducing the number of keywords or using a more general word instead of a very specific one (for example, "breast cancer" instead of "lobular carcinoma").

If you want to focus your search, either because hundreds of titles were returned or because you didn't find enough articles that interested you, you have four main options:

1. *Use more, and more specific, keywords.* One way to find out which keywords you might add to narrow your search is to page through some of the hundreds of titles your original set of broad, less specific keywords brought up. Somewhere in the first couple of pages of that large group should be at least one article that sounds similar to what you are looking for. See what words are used in that title or abstract that further define your question, and add those words to your search.

2. *Use restrictive words.* If you page through the first few titles and see a common word or phrase that has nothing to do with what you want, you can filter those articles out. For example, one of the main causes of a condition called lymphedema (swelling of an arm or leg due to problems in the lymphatic system) is removal of lymph nodes after breast cancer surgery. Nine out of ten articles about lymphedema will refer to this situation. But what if you are a man who has lymphedema in your leg because of colon cancer? All those breast cancer articles don't pertain to your situation. In the search bar, type: lymphedema NOT "breast cancer." (The NOT needs to be in all capital letters, otherwise the program will search for the word *not* as a keyword!) This will return all articles about lymphedema that do not pertain to breast cancer. You could also add a more limiting "and" restriction, as in: lymphedema AND "colon cancer." This will return a much smaller set of titles, ones that pertain only to lymphedema and colon cancer.

While this might be a good way to start narrowing down the search, it may eliminate other interesting lymphedema treatment articles that don't mention any cancer. Try different restricting options and see which work best for your condition.

3. *Use the "Related Articles" option.* Once you find an article that is close to what you need, click on "Related Articles" found on the right side of the screen. The program will search for articles that are similar to that article and give you a whole new list. This basically allows you to say to the computer, "That's what I want, get me more like that one." And it will. You can do this from any article. And don't worry, you can always get back to the previous list by clicking on the "Back" button on your browser's tool bar.

4. *Impose limits on the search.* Under the MEDLINE search bar is the word *Limits* with a box next to it. Click on the word *Limits* and another level of detail will be revealed. You will be presented with several choices as to how you would like MEDLINE to choose the articles it pulls up. They are pretty self-explanatory, but in a nutshell, your choices can be "Limited to":

- *All Fields:* Leave this box alone. If you later become proficient with MEDLINE, you can go back and use specific fields to search, such as "Author Name," "Journal Name," "Text Word," "Title Word," or special Medical Subject Heading (MeSH) terms.

- *Only items with abstracts:* If you click on the empty box in front of this phrase, a check mark will appear indicating that you don't want to see titles of articles for which the abstracts are not available. You may miss a couple of interesting articles this way, but without the abstract, you'll have to track them all down individually to know what they are really about. It's up to you if this is worth your time.

- *Publication types:* With this field limiter you can choose to see only Review Articles, Meta-analyses, Randomized Controlled Trials, and Clinical Trials. This can be extremely valuable for an initial search, to cut right to more solid research conclusions by reading only reviews or meta-analyses.

- *Language:* This lets you choose to find articles printed only in a particular language. Although many fine studies are performed in other countries, you may wish to restrict your search to English if you plan to read the original text. (All abstracts included in MEDLINE are translated into English, so you can always read a summary of foreign studies.)

- *Subsets:* Don't change this setting. If you become proficient at using MEDLINE, you can browse some of the subsets, which give a more limited number of results based on a smaller population of articles.

- *Ages:* Unless you are very concerned about finding only articles that deal with a certain age group, there is no reason to change this. It can be helpful, however, for limiting the search only to pediatric studies or only adult studies.

- *Human or animal:* If you find yourself presented with a lot of animal studies from your search, you can choose "Human" and pull up only articles that studied people.

- *Gender:* If it is important to you, you can choose to select studies that included only female or only male subjects. There is rarely a need to do this, however, unless you are looking for something very exceptional, such as studies of men with breast cancer.

- *Entrez date:* This is the date that entries have been added to this MEDLINE database. It won't be important unless you do frequent searches and don't want to pull up articles you've already seen. In that case, you can set a limit, such as "60 Days," which will tell MEDLINE to find articles that have been added to the database within only the past two months.

- *Publication date—From year   month   day To year   month day:* This allows you to limit your search based on the date of the publication. For example, you can stipulate that you want to see only articles that have been published in the past two years, or between January and March of last year.

Once you've set your limits and have typed your keywords into the search bar at the top of the page, simply click "Go" to start the limited search. You'll notice that the little box next to "Limits" on the next Web page has a check mark in it, signifying that it recognized that you are using limits. To eliminate the limits, simply click on the checked box to remove the check.

MISCELLANEOUS TIPS

• A wonderful feature of PubMed is the ability to have the computer track your search. As long as you keep moving and don't let the computer sit idle for an hour, you can click on *"History"* under the search bar at the top of the page. It will list out all the keywords you used, what limits were imposed, and how many articles were retrieved in that search. Clicking on that number (on the right side of the screen) will take you back to the results of that search. Print your search history after each MEDLINE session and add it to your Personal Health Log. You can refer back to this sheet later to remember what keywords were most valuable, or where you left off in your search.

• To *print* any page, use the print feature on your browser. There is no special MEDLINE print feature.

• You can get the full articles from a medical library or consumer health library (see chapter 5). It's also possible to set up an account with a local medical library through a service called *Loansome Doc*, which allows you to order articles that will be delivered to you at home by fax or mail. Basically, you set up an account, send a check to the library liaison to secure your account, and then order documents through the MEDLINE site. The cost of this service varies, but generally ranges from $10 to $20 per article retrieved and sent. Order carefully since you will not be able to return the article if it's not what you thought it was. To set up an account, or order once your account is set up, put an article on the clipboard (see box above). Then, click on the word *Clipboard* underneath the search bar at the top of the page. On the bar just above the name of the article, you'll see several command buttons, including one that reads "Order." Click on the "Order" button. A new page will come up that allows you to sign in if you have already set up an account, or to find out more about Loansome Doc if you are a new user.

Follow the directions for "If you are new . . ." to set up an account. Setting up an account takes several days, so if you've found articles you'd like to order, make sure you print out the titles so you can find them easily once your account is active.

SOME HELPFUL HINTS WHEN USING MEDLINE

- You can search on an *author's name* by typing it into the search box. The form MEDLINE uses is "Lastname Initial Initial," for example Dooley WC (no punctuation marks). If you don't know the initials, the last name will do. You can also combine a name search with another keyword to further narrow the results in case the doctor you are searching has a common name. For example, "Dooley WC" AND "breast cancer."
- You can use a *"wild card"* when searching MEDLINE. For searches in which several similar words can be used, an asterisk (*) will stand in for the unwritten letters. For example, if you write "carcin*" you'll retrieve all words that start with the letters "carcin" with any ending. So carcin* will retrieve "carcinogen," "carcinogens," "carcinogenic," "carcinogenesis," and "carcinoma."
- You don't have to keep going back to the MEDLINE homepage to start a search. You can put new keywords in the search bar at the top of any page.
- As you become more familiar with MEDLINE searches, read some of the additional resource information and FAQs found on the left side of the MEDLINE homepage screen. You'll learn about other, more intricate ways of searching, and will have answers to problems you may have run into along the way.

▶ ACTION PLAN

1. Go to medical journals last, after you've sought out other sources of information and understand the basics of your disease.
2. Don't change your behavior or get worried and upset because of information presented in a single study; how-

ever, if you see similar information repeatedly, be sure to discuss your concerns with your doctor.

3. Read as much or as little of the article as makes sense for you. The goal is to understand the study and what it means, not become an expert on statistics.

4. If you have concerns or questions about a particular study, talk with your doctor.

5. If an article seems appropriate for your condition, copy it and put it in your Personal Health Log.

EXAMPLE OF A MEDLINE SEARCH

Let's assume a hypothetical diagnosis of avascular necrosis of the hip, a disorder in which the blood supply to the long bones of the body is cut off and bone starts to die. Our imaginary physician has recommended a hip replacement, and we want to find out what information is in the medical literature. Our questions are: For avascular necrosis, what are the latest advancements in hip replacement? Are there any other treatment options?

Our potential keywords are "avascular necrosis," "hip," "hip replacement," "treatment," and "alternatives."

Just to see how popular a subject it is, let's use only the keywords "avascular necrosis" to start. And since we want to know the *latest advances,* let's limit the results only to articles published in the past year. Type "avascular necrosis" on the search bar, then click on the word *Limits* under the search bar at the top of the page. Next to "Publication Date," type in the dates that make about a one-year period. (This doesn't have to be exact, just plugging in the years will do.) Click on the "Go" button.

We find that there are more than a hundred articles about avascular necrosis (AVN) published in the past year. We definitely need to narrow the field. As you scan down the titles, look to see if any topics seem particularly inappropriate. Here, there are articles on AVN of joints other than the hip that we don't need, and quite a few on children. To eliminate these, we will add another keyword in the search bar—"hip"—then click on "Limits" and choose "All adult: 19+ years" on the "AGE" pull-down. Make these changes, then click on "Go."

Bingo! The number of articles with adult subjects published in the past year that fit the keywords "avascular necrosis hip" is narrowed to under thirty. This is very manageable and, supposedly, exactly what we want to read. (Actual numbers may differ, depending on the years searched.)

Types of Scientific Studies

Scientists use different methods for gathering information. The type of study used generally depends on the kind of information available, the question that needs to be answered, and whether or not an experiment can be used to isolate and test a hypothesis (versus observing natural conditions as they occur). The following are the most common types of studies you'll find.

RANDOMIZED CONTROLLED TRIAL

These are experiments designed to find out whether one or more groups have different outcomes if they are given a particular treatment, compared to a "control" group that receives a placebo treatment—one in which the patient believes he or she is receiving a treatment, but really isn't. (Most people have heard about the "sugar pill" placebo, in which patients are given a pill to take that is made up only of sugar or other inactive substance that cannot have a therapeutic effect. Using placebos allows scientists to separate the *real* effects of the treatment from the "placebo effect," in which patients feel better simply because they think they are receiving treatment.)

In a randomized controlled trial, scientists can give one group of patients the medication to be tested, while another group of patients receives only a placebo. After a certain amount of time, the two groups are compared to determine whether the patients in the medication group had an effect that was different from the patients in the placebo group.

It is important to have a placebo group as a control because the effect of suggestion—mind over body—is very powerful. It has been estimated that up to 30 percent of the effect of any medication or treatment is due to the belief that the treatment will work, and that people who receive only a placebo treatment will show up to a 30 percent improvement, even though the treatment wasn't real. A placebo can take many forms. Patients in controlled trials can receive sugar pills, injections that contain only saline or another inert substance, and, in rare cases, placebo surgery, in which the patient is cut open and then sewn shut, but with no actual treatment being done.

In these experiments, it is very important that patients not know which group they are in because that knowledge alone could cause them to respond differently. Often, even the scientists don't know which patients are receiving which treatment. These are called double-blind studies, since both the patient and the doctor are "blind" as to who is getting the real treatment. Double-blind studies are used to eliminate the possibility of a doctor giving subtle clues to the patient about the type of treatment he or she might be getting, or to keep the doctor from acting differently toward the two groups. For example, a doctor who is very excited about a new form of antidepressant might act more cheerful or hopeful in front of the patients getting the medication than in front of the patients receiving the placebo—and that small difference might be enough to make some patients more cheerful or hopeful. The antidepressant effect wouldn't be the effect of the medication then, but the effect of having such a nice doctor.

The other important piece of randomized controlled trials is the "randomized" part. These days, patients are given either the real treatment or the placebo, based on computer-generated randomization procedures. Being randomly assigned to either the treatment or placebo group helps to ensure that the groups being compared are as equal as possible—they are both comprised of the same general mix of people. If they were not randomized, it would be possible for doctors to select patients for a particular group based on subtle differences, such as who might have a more pleasing personality or who is taller, or any number of other characteristics that may or may not affect the outcome of the study. If the patients (or "subjects," as people in experiments are called) are randomized, there is no need to worry about those other extraneous effects, so any effect should be due entirely to the difference in treatment.

Although randomized controlled trials are considered the best kind of study, it's not always possible or even desirable to perform them. What if a doctor wants to set out to prove that a certain chemical causes cancer? He can't give the chemical to some subjects, a placebo to other subjects, and see if the people in the chemical group got more cancer. It's unethical, and no scientist would put people's lives in jeopardy that way. But there are other ways to study these types of difficult questions.

COHORT STUDIES

In cohort studies, the subjects are chosen based on specifically defined differences, with as many other characteristics as possible being identical. For example, the imaginary scientist who wants to prove that a particular chemical causes cancer might compare two groups of people: those who work with the potentially hazardous chemical, and those who have no opportunity for exposure. The scientist would follow these two groups of people over time to see if those in the exposure group got more cancers than those in the nonexposure group. This type of study is less reliable than randomized controlled trials because it's always possible that other factors might account for the difference. For example, if people who work with those types of potentially hazardous materials are of lower socioeconomic status than those who work safer jobs, there may be other factors in their home environment that may also lead them to develop more cancers. The goal is to look at groups as similar as possible to eliminate this kind of bias, although there is no way to totally control for it.

CASE-CONTROL STUDIES

These studies are often used to help determine possible causes or correlates of disease. Patients who have a particular disease or condition are "matched" with people who do not have the disease. (They are matched on as many important characteristics as possible, such as sex or economic status.) Then, other data are gathered, either from medical records or by interview, and the groups are compared to see what differences in their lifestyle or possible disease exposure might have led one group to get the disease while the other group remained healthy. These types of studies are not as strong as the previous two because the information looked at here is historical, or *retrospective*. The patients already have the disease, so the scientists attempt to look back into their life history to see what might have led to the problem. In contrast, both randomized controlled trials and cohort studies are *prospective*—that is, they look at groups of people over a period of time to determine what will happen in the future, either in terms of treatment results or disease development.

EPIDEMIOLOGIC STUDIES

The field of epidemiology looks at the occurrence and causes of diseases in a population, as opposed to looking at individual patients. Epidemiologic studies can compare large groups of people to determine differences in disease prevalence and spread. For example, when you read that women in Japan have a much lower rate of breast cancer than women in the United States, that is an example of two large groups being compared. Next, the lifestyle differences among the groups might be compared to see what might be different enough to cause the higher rates of cancer in the United States. If a possible source of cancer is found in the United States (or a source of protection from cancer is found in Japan), then smaller experimental studies can look more specifically at these factors to determine if they do, indeed, cause or protect against cancer.

CASE REPORTS

These are medical histories of a single patient followed for a particular period of time. Case reports are the least informative form of a study, but they are often used to illustrate an example of a particular disease or treatment, or to provide possible clues about a disease for which further research would be needed.

READING A CITATION

There is a standard way that medical citations on journal articles are listed.

1. Names of the authors of the article. Each name is listed surname first, followed by that scientist's initials. If a large number of scientists contributed, you may see only one or two names, followed by "et al.," which basically means "and everyone else."
2. Title of the article.
3. Title of the journal in which the article appeared. This will often be abbreviated. You can look up journal abbreviations on Index Medicus, available online at www.medscape.com/Home/Search/Index Medicus/IndexMedicus.htm.
4. The date of publication.
5. The volume and issue number of the journal in which the article was printed, usually seen in the form of "volume (issue number)." Journals are often bound together in large books for storage in libraries. These numbers help identify the exact article.
6. Pages on which the article appeared.

For example:

Doe JR, Smith CA, Lawrence TM. How to Understand a Journal Article. *J Pers Examp.* August 2001;806(1):1956-1958.

10. Other Information Sources

THERE are seemingly endless sources of health information. Here are guidelines for finding and evaluating some of the more common ones.

Magazines

In general, magazines are fine for prevention and wellness information. Look for disease-specific magazines to help manage illness.

If the only places you've ever looked for magazines were your grocery store or book shop, then you haven't even begun to appreciate the full range of health magazines available. There are four main categories of magazines that can provide health information:

GENERAL INTEREST, MASS MARKET MAGAZINES
These contain a mix of articles on home, family, entertainment, cooking, gardening, and health. The titles are familiar: *Family Circle*, *Glamour*, *Good Housekeeping*, *Ladies' Home Journal*, *Parade*, *Reader's Digest*, *Redbook*, *Self*, and *Woman's Day*. While you wouldn't turn to these magazines primarily for health informa-

tion, you may run across an interesting article while you're looking for a new chicken recipe. Should you trust it? Like newspapers and television shows, these magazines are highly concerned with sensational stories that can easily capture the reader's interest. Because magazine writers have more time in which to do interviews and research than newspaper writers, the information provided is often accurate and useful. However, it can be incomplete due to space restrictions or biased due to advertiser concerns. Further, many articles contain real-life stories of people who have suffered from the disorder being discussed. Because of the need to be instantly interesting, these stories are often not typical for the disease, and may be frightening. Ignore the stories, but use any information as a jumping-off point for your own research. Note any physicians who gave opinions you feel might be helpful to you in the future. These publications are available at supermarkets, bookstores, and newsstands. Many have websites, and some will allow you to search archives or read articles online.

NEWS MAGAZINES

The big three—*Time, Newsweek,* and *U.S. News & World Report*— are usually highly trustworthy sources of information. Although you wouldn't make them your number one spot to search for health information, these magazines print at least one health column each week, and often larger full-length health articles. They strive for accuracy and try to present a complete picture of the issue, but again, space constraints sometimes force them to gloss over certain facts. Thanks to the tremendous resources and the prestige of these magazines, the physicians quoted are usually top-notch, and the graphics are clear and easy to understand. Because they, too, are concerned with sales, these magazines focus on the more common disorders, especially cancer and heart disease, but there are often stories about breakthroughs in other areas. Each of these magazines also has a website where you can search the archives and read articles online. Be forewarned: You'll have to wade through quite a number of irrelevant titles to find the information you want, since, for example, if you search for the word *arthritis*, you'll not only get articles on arthritis, but every article that mentions that a particular person has arthritis or phrases containing the word *arthritis*.

For *Time*—http://www.time.com.
For *Newsweek*—http://www.newsweek.com.
For *U.S. News & World Report*—http://www.usnews.com.

MASS MARKET HEALTH MAGAZINES

These magazines specialize in wellness, prevention, and fitness topics, with occasional information about specific diseases. Some focus on exercise and diet, and are therefore less useful for people dealing with a condition. The best of the prevention and wellness genre are *Prevention* and *Health*, which provide fact-checked information in an easy-to-read style. Again, these magazines need to attract your attention, so there are occasional scare-tactic titles, such as "When Worrying Becomes Deadly," but they also publish valuable information on how to prevent heart attacks or the latest breast biopsy information. Since these magazines are aimed more at the general, healthy public, there is less disease-specific information. But if you want to learn the basics of good health, these magazines may be right for you. They are available at supermarkets, bookstores, and newsstands. One interesting development in the mass-market health magazine field is the publication *MAMM*, which was launched October 1997. This magazine is written to meet the needs of women diagnosed with breast and reproductive cancers. It is the first magazine to "mainstream" a disease, and includes medical articles, information on alternative therapies, and inspirational stories. It is available in some bookstores and newsstands. Visit the website at http://www.mamm.com for information on how to subscribe.

DISEASE-SPECIFIC MAGAZINES

Although there are not many such magazines published, they are very helpful resources, providing up-to-date information about treatments, inspiration, and resources. The best are typically supported or endorsed by national associations, such as *Arthritis Today* by the Arthritis Foundation, *Diabetes Advisor* and *Diabetes Forecast* by the American Diabetes Association, and *Inside MS* by the National Multiple Sclerosis Society. These are only available by subscription, although many can be read online. Call or check the website of an appropriate organization to see if they publish a magazine or newsletter (see "Newsletters" below). A more general but highly accurate magazine is *FDA Consumer*, the official magazine of the Food and Drug Administration (FDA). Along with FDA news, such as new drug approvals and updates, there are full-length articles on specific diseases, prevention, and other health concerns. It is available from the Superintendent of Documents, U.S. Printing Office, or online at http://www.fda.gov/fdac, where you can also read selected articles.

Newsletters

Newsletters are very useful sources of health information. There are several fine health and wellness newsletters, and a wide selection of excellent disease-related ones.

Newsletters are minimagazines, usually without the advertisements. They are generally between eight and sixteen pages long, and can be either general or disease-specific. The best newsletters are associated with or published by a major university or national disease organization. Those that aren't should have an advisory board of physicians and specialists (which would be listed in the staff box somewhere in the newsletter). Although they vary in appearance (from plain paper with no illustrations or photographs to heavier, high-quality paper with full-color illustration), don't use how they look as a measure of quality—they are all generally well-researched, accurate sources of information. Since they each have a slightly different focus and style, choose the one that suits you and your needs best.

General health newsletters provide articles on a broad range of topics, from specific disease information to nutrition, exercise, prevention, weight loss, pharmaceuticals, new medical procedures, and a question-and-answer section. They are available only by subscription. If you are interested in subscribing, most companies will send a free sample newsletter for you to evaluate. Many have Internet sites that tell you how to subscribe or sign up for your sample issue (see chapter 8 for Internet information). Among the best: *Harvard Health Letter* (there is also a *Harvard Men's Health Watch* and *Harvard Women's Health Watch*), *Health News* (from the publishers of the *New England Journal of Medicine*), *Johns Hopkins Medical Letter: Health After 50; Mayo Clinic Health Letter, Nutrition Action Health Letter, Tufts University Health & Nutrition Letter, University of California-Berkeley Wellness Letter*, and *Women's Health Advisor* (affiliated with Cornell University).

Disease-specific newsletters can provide a substantial amount of focused information to patients, and should definitely be considered as an ongoing information resource for anyone with a chronic disease. There is a newsletter for nearly every disease or disease category. Once you understand your condition, a good newsletter can keep you apprised of the latest useable information by condensing medical studies and FDA news into about ten pages of easy-to-read text. Again, look for those that are affiliated with or published by reputable universities or national disease organizations—call or check their websites to see if they have a newsletter they endorse. Some newsletters are available only by subscription, while others are available at no cost online.

Disease Associations/Organizations

Legitimate associations provide some of the best information available.

Specific disease associations act as information resources for people diagnosed with that disease, and the information is usually provided free or at minimal cost. Much of the information is available online, but if you don't have access to the Internet you can always call the organization and ask them to mail what you need.

There is an association or organization for just about every disease, either in government (see chapter 7) or the public sector. For some diseases, such as breast or prostate cancer, there are several. Since the entire purpose of these organizations is to fight their adopted disease, they have a tight focus on exactly the topic that interests you. Take advantage of all they have to offer. Because the best associations have physician advisory boards, their information is usually highly accurate.

One problem you may have is with potentially bogus associations or foundations. There are some unscrupulous people who create organizations with names that are remarkably similar to the names of legitimate organizations. For example, the American Cancer Society is a well-respected, authoritative organization, but it is not the same as the "National Cancer Society" or the "American Cancer Association." The National Health Information Center (NHIC) is a government agency whose job it is to put you in touch with organizations that can answer your health questions. If you visit their website or call the office they will refer you to the best associations for your disorder and provide you with toll-free telephone numbers for those associations. This takes some of the guesswork out of knowing which associations are legitimate and which are a waste of time. The NHIC can be reached through the Internet at http://www.health.gov/nhic or by telephone at 1-800-336-4797 (toll free) or 301-565-4167 (local). If an organization is not on this list, examine it much more carefully before donating money or using any information obtained from them. (The NHIC claims that listing an organization does not imply endorsement by the government, but their list does appear to exclude known copycat or disreputable sites.)

Friends and Family

Friends and family members may prove to be valuable sources of support and firsthand knowledge. They can lead you to other patients or doctors to contact. But be wary of disease horror stories, anecdotal cures, and rumors.

Although we tend to take our friends and family for granted and rarely think of them as sources of information, many doctors see tremendous value in enlisting their help. "We ask patients to talk to friends who have had similar procedures," says Forrest Lang, M.D., of East Tennessee State University. "That should be encouraged rather than discouraged. . . . People will tell you what has worked for them. If a procedure is good, most people's experiences are going to be good."

So talk to friends and family about what their experiences were like with similar surgeries or medications. Learn what they already know firsthand—with the emphasis on *firsthand*. You don't need to hear the rumors or horror stories of what happened to Aunt Millie's second cousin's friend, or what they think happened to their next-door neighbor. If they start to tell these kinds of stories, interrupt and ask if they have the neighbor's phone number so you can call him or her directly to get the story firsthand.

You can also ask friends and family to assist in your information search. Use them as an extension of yourself, since you can't do everything at once. The next time people ask if there is anything they can do, in addition to asking for a ride to your next doctor's appointment, send them to the library or the bookstore, or ask them to do an online search for you on a specific topic, or let them call a consumer health library to request information—anything that will not need your constant supervision so as to free up your time for more complex searches.

Videotapes and Audiotapes

Videotapes and audiotapes are a mixed bag.

It is very important not to get sucked into just any health videotape or audiotape. These media can be quite compelling. Actually seeing someone speak to you, hearing the voice that may be quite earnest and convincing, is valuable only if the information is accurate. Otherwise, it's just another TV show.

Look for videos and audiotapes that are endorsed or produced by a major university or disease organization. This will ensure that the material has been seen and evaluated by professionals who are putting their reputations on the line. Don't bother with any disease-specific or treatment-oriented video or audiotape that is more than two years old—the information will likely be outdated. Ask your doctor or the librarian at a consumer health library (see chapter 5) to recommend videos, and see if you can borrow them—they can be very expensive to purchase and will become obsolete quickly.

One source that has highly accurate and highly relevant videotapes is Health Dialog. In conjunction with the reputable Foundation for Informed Decision Making, this company sells videotapes on a select group of topics (although the company claims the number of titles will grow over the next few years). Specific topics are especially relevant to people with prostate disease, breast cancer, uterine conditions, low-back pain, hypertension, and ischemic heart disease. Of added interest are the videos dealing with Advance Directives (how to make end-of-life decisions and achieve peace of mind) and Shared Decisions (how to choose among various treatment options). These are reviewed quarterly and updated as needed, so they are always current. The biggest drawback is the price: $250 per video, but if you are facing life-altering decisions, this cost may be worth it for these top-of-the-line products. Contact Health Dialog at 617-854-7440, or see their website at www.healthdialog.com.

Review Reports

Excellent as a year-in-review, but they cover only the most common diseases or health areas.

Some companies scan the literature for specific disease information and publish yearly update reports of varying lengths.

The most comprehensive reports are the *Johns Hopkins White Papers*, which provide quite a lot of information in about sixty to eighty-five pages. Reviewed by top physicians at Johns Hopkins University School of Medicine, these annual tomes include reprinted medical journal articles, how current research might translate into treatment options, drug update information, case studies, and bibliographies—all written for the serious information gatherer. Topics covered change year to year depending on how well they sell, but the most popular and likely to be continued are Arthritis, Coronary Heart Disease, Depression and Anxiety, Diabetes Mellitus, Hypertension and Stroke, Low-Back Pain and Osteoporosis, Prostate Disorders, and Vision. Breast Cancer is slated to be added beginning in 2001. These can be ordered for $19.95 (plus shipping and handling) at 1-800-829-0422.

Another well-respected review series is *Well-Connected*, published by Nidus Information Services. These patient information booklets are much shorter, generally less than ten pages, and published quarterly. They are reviewed by an editorial board at Harvard Medical School and Massachusetts General Hospital, so their accuracy is virtually guaranteed. Although less information is provided than the *Johns Hopkins White Papers*, more diseases and topics are covered (approximately one hundred at last count). For $29, individuals can order a subscription to all the reports for one full year. To see available reports and order online, go to their website at http://www.well-connected.com, or call 1-800-334-9355.

For-Fee Information Providers

These may be worth the cost for serious or rare diseases.

There are some companies that will do a health information search specifically for you, for a fee. Some people have these providers do an initial search and then take over from there; others use the service instead of doing their own search. What's best for you depends on your personality and needs. If you need a lot of information in a hurry and feel that you aren't up to the task yourself, many of these companies can provide a lot of valuable information quickly. But there's nothing they can do that you can't do as well, it's just that they've had a little more practice at it. In fact, many of these companies were started by people who had severe illnesses themselves and had to learn how to do health searches on their own. (And remember, consumer health libraries can and will do many of the same searches at no cost—see chapter 5.)

The way these services work is that you either speak with a researcher or fill out an application form specifying your disorder, health condition, and the precise information you want to know. In some cases, the researcher will help you narrow down the questions that are relevant to you. Researchers then work to put together an individualized report, created just for you.

There are several for-fee information providers out there, with varying levels of quality and performance. The best known and probably oldest company is The Health Resource, Inc. In about three to five business days they will provide you with a bound, individualized research report that includes all treatment options, new research, outstanding specialists for your disorder, support organizations, and self-help measures. Their reports on noncancer conditions cost $275 (plus shipping), and cancer reports cost $375 (plus shipping). Best of all, there is a thirty-day money-back guarantee if you are dissatisfied for any reason. They can be contacted at 1-800-949-0090, or see their website at http://www.thehealthresource.com.

Choosing a health information provider can be difficult. There are an increasing number of them, and there is no absolute standard for how to assess them, short of actually looking at a completed report. Some guidelines:

Look for a money-back guarantee: Some offer it, some don't. You can be sure that a company that offers to give you your money back if you're dissatisfied won't stay in business long if they don't produce quality goods.

Look at the Web address: The Web address should be similar to the name of the company. This isn't a foolproof method of finding a good company, but it's one rule of thumb for weeding out inexperienced ones. The URL for The Health Resource is www.thehealthresource.com. The name is in the URL. Avoid companies that start with "geocities" or other intermediary names. They are most likely less experienced and possibly underfunded.

Look at the website: Again, not a foolproof method, but you can get a feel for the company by its site. Does it look amateurish? Does it lack information? Does it use cartoon characters as illustrations? If yes, then skip it and try another. Does it look professional? Does it give a sample report? Does it fully explain the services and price? If yes to these, you might want to look further.

Look at what is offered in the report: Some companies provide only the results of an Internet search, while others give you names of physicians, alternative medicine information, or patient success stories. Granted, the more you get, the higher the price will be, but make sure you're at least getting what you expect.

Check the pricing: Some companies, such as The Health Resource, Inc., give standard prices for their reports. Others charge by the hour. It is not in a patient's best interest to sign up with an hourly rate company because if you have a complex problem (or a slow researcher), you may end up spending far more than you bargained for.

Call the company: Once you settle on one or two companies that fit your needs, call and talk to them about your problem. This will give you a feel for how professional they are, how well they understand your problem, and how comfortable you feel. Ask questions like how long they have been in business, how their researchers are trained, and how the company got started. Compare the companies and choose the one you feel most satisfied with.

Brochures and Pamphlets

These provide only basic and minimal information, but they're still worth reading.

Because doctors have such limited time, they need to find quick ways to explain basic disease and treatment information to their patients. Many of them choose brochures and pamphlets for this purpose. Chances are you've picked up one or two already. These are fine sources for very basic information, and they are often written in a way that everyone can understand, regardless of how much familiarity one has with medical terminology.

Look for them in your doctor's office, and take two or three with you—one for yourself, and a couple to hand out to the people who need to understand your disorder, such as a spouse, a child, or a friend. Some brochures and pamphlets are available from government sources (see chapter 7) or from specific disease organizations. Call the organization or look on their website to see if they print brochures. These are often free of charge.

Caregivers

11. Doctors

IF you've been diagnosed with a medical condition, chances are you're going to have to deal with more than one doctor. You'll keep the primary doctor you've always used, then perhaps add a specialist or two to treat and monitor your condition, and perhaps a surgeon, a radiologist, an anesthesiologist. These people will hold your life in their hands at various points during your treatment. They are your partners in health, your medical guides, the people with whom you discuss your most private bodily functions. They see you naked, inside and out.

So why is it that many of us spend more time trying to find a decent car mechanic than we do locating good doctors?

Part of the answer has to do with the legacy of paternalism in medicine. Most of us grew up believing that doctors were all-knowing and infallible, at least when it came to making medical decisions. "People want to trust their doctors more than they necessarily want to trust their car mechanics," says Timothy B. McCall, M.D., internist and author of "Examining Your Doctor" (available free of charge on www.DrMcCall.com). "When people are sick, they often are in a vulnerable position. They want to believe that [their doctor] has their best interests in mind."

If that were true, then all doctors would be equally good and it wouldn't matter which one you choose. The doctor down the street would be just as good as, but more convenient than, the one from Massachusetts General, the Mayo Clinic, Johns Hopkins, UCLA, Duke, Stanford, Memorial Sloan-Kettering, or any of the other famous medical centers and hospitals.

But it isn't true. Not all doctors were educated the same, not all doctors have the same personality, not all doctors are equally skilled, not all doctors have equal knowledge.

"In many ways, the primary determinant of the quality of care you're going to get is the quality of the physician," says Dr. Timothy McCall. "People think you just go to the doctor, and the doctor does the right thing. They don't understand what tremendous variability there is, not just in the quality of doctors but in their practice styles."

So it is vitally important that you spend some time choosing the right primary care physician and the specialists who will be directly treating your condition.

Even when you're healthy, having a good and trusted primary care physician (PCP) is important. This is the doctor who will be your partner, the person who will act as the gatekeeper and hub of all your medical care. When you are well, this doctor will recommend ways to keep you healthy. And if you become ill, a trusted PCP can help you choose good medical treatments and coordinate future care.

PCPs can handle routine care and minor illnesses just fine. But when you're diagnosed with a serious illness, you're going to want to see a specialist. Specialists have extra training and are board certified as experts in specific disease areas. There are even specialists among specialists—surgeons are specialists, but there are also highly specialized surgeons who operate only on a specific area of the body, such as the breast, hand, or brain. Specialists are better at treating serious diseases because they have more training and experience; and since they have a more focused area of expertise, they know more about the latest medical treatments and procedures.

Studies have shown that having a specialist treat your condition may save your life. A published review of the literature found that specialists were more likely to use medications associated with improved survival, to recommend routine screening, to use more diagnostic tests, and sometimes to have better outcomes. For example, a study by researchers at Duke University found that heart attack patients who were admitted to a hospital by a cardiologist (a specialist) were 12 percent less likely to die in the next year than patients who were admitted by a PCP, presumably due to better heart care.

And treatment by specialists may even be cost-effective, which will be an important consideration for health maintenance organizations in the future. One study looked at the different costs associated with having patients hospitalized for diabetic ketoacidosis (a condition that can result in coma or death if untreated). Patients who were regularly treated by a diabetes specialist had shorter hospital stays, a lower readmission rate, and in general cost less to treat than patients who were typically treated by a PCP.

So you'll need to choose your PCP and specialists with care. But what about the other physicians you may see? Some people also recommend doing a background check of every doctor who has anything to do with your care, including anesthesiologists and radiologists. If that seems like a chore, John D. Birkmeyer, M.D., assistant professor of surgery at Dartmouth Medical School in New Hampshire, agrees. "I think it would be an unrealistic and fairly onerous burden to place on individual patients to have to check out the certifications and the resources at every single level." Instead, he and other experts recommend going to a busy, high-volume hospital where all team members are likely to have lots of experience with your type of illness or surgery. (See chapter 12 for more information on how to choose a good hospital.)

Choosing the Right Doctor

If you want to find the best doctors for you, it's going to take time, persistence, a few phone calls, perhaps an Internet search, interviews, and a little soul-searching, but it will be worth it to have the piece of mind of knowing you are well cared-for. Of course, not all illnesses will allow the luxury of time to search out the right physician. If you are in the middle of having a heart attack, you're not going to be able to pick and choose which doctor you want to treat you. In that case, you have to trust that you'll be treated well in the closest emergency room, and that your carefully chosen primary care physician will oversee your immediate recovery. Once you are back on your feet, you can search for the best cardiologist for you.

There are a few factors to consider as you begin searching for a PCP or specialist.

Travel comfort zone: Some people are willing to travel hundreds of miles to be treated by one of the country's top specialists; others are less willing to travel, either because of physical limitations, financial constraints, or for reasons of convenience. Decide for yourself how far you are willing to travel to see a primary care physician, and how far you are willing to travel to see any specialists you may need. These distances may very well be different. PCPs are usually seen more frequently, and often for semi-emergency acute illnesses, so you may want to have that doctor be relatively nearby. Your comfort zone may also differ depending on the illness your specialist is treating.

How *NOT* to choose doctors

- From the telephone book
- From an advertisement on television or in a magazine or newspaper
- From paid listings in doctor databases
- Because they are "nice"
- Because they were the only ones to say that there was "nothing wrong" with you
- Because they write prescriptions easily, sometimes without examining you
- Because they give free samples of prescription drugs

Chronic management of a relatively benign disease can usually be handled well by local specialists. But if you have a life-threatening, dangerous, or rare illness, you may be willing to travel great distances to be treated in one of "the best" medical centers (see chapter 12).

Your insurance: Depending on the type and level of health insurance you have, your choices may be limited. Some provide lists of participating physicians who are considered part of their "network," and if you choose from that list, your medical care costs will be minimal. Others allow you to choose your own physician. Some allow you to see physicians outside the "network," but require you to pay a percentage of the costs. Others won't cover nonaffiliated physician visits at all. Find out in advance what the scope and limitations of your insurance are so that you can choose the best care you can afford. (If you are willing to pay out-of-pocket for some medical expenses, determine how much you are willing to spend.)

Hospital preferences: Physicians are usually affiliated with only one or two hospitals. If you are fortunate enough to have several good hospitals to choose from in your area, decide which hospital you feel is best for you (see chapter 12). Then call the hospital to get a list of the appropriate specialists or PCPs who have affiliations there. If your hospital choices are limited, decide how far you are willing to travel to see a doctor affiliated with the highest quality hospital within a decent driving range.

Medical groups: In this era of managed care, it is becoming increasingly difficult to find individual doctors in private practice. Many PCPs band together in medical groups that can vary in size from two to twelve or more. The benefits are that the office hours are usually extended (some are open 365 days a year) and appointments are easier to get, especially on short notice. Also, the doctors may support each other. "Doctors who work together can trade notes with each other, share information, get what they call 'curb-side consult'—just bump into someone in the hall and say, I've got this patient, what do you think," says Dr. Timothy McCall. "That can be quite a useful thing. It's a way for doctors to keep up-to-date. It's a way for doctors to interact with specialists under the same roof and learn from them in a way they might not otherwise be able to." The main drawback is that there is no guarantee you'll see the same physician each time you visit, and therefore continuity of care may be compromised. Granted, your medical chart is kept current in the office, but you may still end up having to explain your problem over and over again to different physicians. If medical groups are your only option, follow the guidelines below for choosing one doctor from the group that you would like to see primarily, then try to schedule any nonemergency appointments with that doctor.

Other important factors: Some women prefer to see only women doctors for gynecologic problems, some patients prefer to be treated by doctors who have been practicing for more than twenty years, some patients want a physician who is knowledgeable about alternative and complementary therapies, and some patients require greater flexibility in office hours. Write down a list of the things that really matter to you.

Once you know the answers to these guiding factors, you can begin searching for the best physician *for you*. It's important to realize that there is no single *best* physician or specialist. The one who's best for you may not be the best one for your mother, or your child, or your neighbor. The goal is to make an informed choice, to decide for yourself who will work to help you become the healthiest person you can be. (If you already have a PCP and/or specialist, you can use many of the same steps to review how good a health partner that physician is for you.)

STEP 1: GATHER NAMES

If you ask enough people which physician they would recommend, the names of some of the best doctors will keep popping up. The medical community is, in some ways, like a small town—and just as in a small town, everyone seems to know everyone else's reputation and business. Although doctors will rarely come right out and tell you which physicians to avoid, they are usually very happy to refer people to good-quality doctors. And nonphysicians always have opinions about who the best doctors are. Make a list of all the names you gather. Highlight those names that keep reappearing.

• Start by asking friends and family for recommendations. For every name they give you, ask why they like that particular doctor. If you are looking for a specialist, ask if they know anyone who has your same illness, then find out if that person is happy with his or her doctor.

• Ask your current PCP for specialist recommendations and ask specialists for PCP recommendations. (Don't ask your current PCP for a referral to a different PCP unless you are moving and your old PCP would be too far away—it's not tactful and chances are you won't get a decent referral.) Ask your dentist, chiropractor, optometrist, or any other health professional for recommendations.

• Call the appropriate medical department of your local medical school for a specialist referral in your area.

• If you are bold enough, walk into your hospital of choice, go to the department where they treat your type of illness, and ask the nurses on staff for physician recommendations. Nurses have some of the best insights since they have seen these doctors under all conditions. (If the department seems busy, ask when some of the lighter times are and come back then. You won't get a thoughtful referral from a nurse who's busy doing her job.)

• Look on the Internet for doctors who specialize in your disease, either on university websites (see chapter 8) or nonprofit disease association websites (see chapter 10). Also, look on MEDLINE to see which physicians have published extensively or have written recent review articles about your disease (see chapter 9). Also, look for doctors who have written books about your illness. If these doctors are not in your area and if you are willing to travel, add these names to your list. If you are not willing to travel, it may be possible to contact these doctors for a referral to a highly qualified doctor in your area. If the highly cited doctor you find is in your area already, highlight that name as a good potential.

Once you have this list of names, check to see how many fit your initial checklist in terms of distance, insurance coverage, and other qualities. (Remember, it will be rare to find one physician who fits all criteria and has gotten good reports from everyone. For example, all doctors have patients who die despite the best medical care. But if the person who died was a friend, you will be less likely to rate that doctor highly.) Take all the information you gather, note which physicians meet much of your criteria, and then go on to Step 2.

If you don't have any names that fit your needs, which can happen if you live in a remote location or if your insurance coverage is limited, then you might have to work in reverse from what you have. Start with a list of names of all the doctors in your area or who are covered by your insurance, then ask everyone you know if they know reasons why you shouldn't go to those physicians. Make your own cuts based on distance, convenience, or other personal factors, then take the names that remain and move on to Step 2.

STEP 2: CHECK THEM OUT

You're going to want to make sure that the doctors who treat you have had appropriate training and good qualifications.

Medical training: Every once in a while you'll read stories of people who were treated (or mistreated) by so-called doctors who didn't have a medical degree. Don't let this happen to you. For all the doctors on your list, find out where they went to medical school, where they did their residency training, and how long they have been practicing. U.S. medical schools are generally considered the best in the world, and they are most likely to keep up with fast-changing technology; therefore, many experts recommend looking for a U.S.-trained physician. Also, as you'll read in chapter 12, busy high-volume hospitals offer the best treatments because doctors there get lots of practice, so look for physicians who did their residency training at a large hospital. (In fact, this information may be even more important than where the doctor went to medical school!) As far as time in practice, there are pros and cons for each possibility: Younger doctors don't have as much experience as older doctors, but they have more recent training and therefore may be more comfortable with newer technology, techniques, and medications. Older doctors, on the other hand, may be better diagnosticians because of their experience. The best place to find this information is on the Internet. Use *AMA Physician Select*, the online doctor finder service of the American Medical Association (http://www.ama-assn.org/aps/amahg.htm). Follow the instructions on the screen to get a full read-out of this information for each doctor. You can also call the doctors' offices directly and ask the office staff.

Board certification: Specialists should be board certified in their area of specialty. That may sound obvious, but there are, for example, physicians who are board certified in dermatology who practice plastic surgery. They can claim to be "board certified," but that doesn't make them plastic surgery specialists. "There are only about 40,000 to 45,000 board-certified general surgeons in the country," says William C. Dooley, M.D., surgical oncologist and director of the Johns Hopkins Breast Center. "But there are over 300,000 people who call themselves surgeons who are not certified." At a minimum, board-certified specialists must undergo additional training and take a written examination of competency in their area. To check board certification of any physician, contact the American Board of Medical Specialties (ABMS) (847-491-9091, or on the Internet at http://www.abms.org). Don't have faith in any "certification" that has not been verified by the ABMS. There are some certificates from sound-alike organizations that can be obtained simply by paying for them, without additional education or testing.

Disciplinary action: Doctors are human. They make mistakes and are subject to the same frailties as the rest of us. While that's understandable, you don't want to entrust your health to incompetent or incapacitated doctors. Doctors can be disciplined for a number of reasons, including alcohol abuse, malpractice, sexual assault, or drug trafficking. To find out if your doctor has had any disciplinary action taken against him or her, or if his or her medical license has been withdrawn, call the medical licensing board for your state. (Call directory assistance for the appropriate number.) You can also go online to the Administrators in Medicine (AIM) DocFinder website (http://www.docboard.org/index.htm). Participating states are linked to this site, and you can look up disciplinary action online.

It's not usually helpful to look at so-called physician "report cards" that claim to rate doctors on various qualities. The ratings can be subjective, which means that the qualities they look for are not necessarily the ones you would want, or there may be commercial interests at stake. "You have to ask yourself who's doing the ratings," says Dr. Timothy McCall. "If a report card is done by, for example, some of these physician referral services, these are often sponsored by a hospital that gets you to use one of their doctors. . . . You're not going to get objective information."

Some report cards may overlook good doctors simply because they don't provide information to the companies that compile the ratings in a form that is easily computerized, and some bad doctors may make the recommendation lists simply because they are well known or because information about their inadequacies is well hidden. Other report cards rate physicians based on the number of patients who die under their care. While this may sound like a valuable piece of information, you can't know if more patients died because the doctor is incompetent or because the doctor is so good that he or she gets the hardest cases, the most severely ill patients (who are generally more likely to die).

"My philosophy," says Dr. Timothy McCall, "is you go as broadly as you can to get information, and then use it all together in coming to your judgment. Don't base everything on one of these lists . . . but pay attention to that . . . use that in your selection process . . . but then use your eyes and ears. Start to pay attention. Start to evaluate."

If you want, you can pay someone to do this search for you. *SearchPointe* will provide background information on any physician licensed to practice in the United States, including medical

school, residency training, specialty certification, licensure information, and records of sanctions or disciplinary actions. They
charge a set fee per physician report. They can be found on the
web at www.searchpointe.com.

Best Doctors will do a more complex search for a higher fee.
This company has compiled a list of highly qualified doctors
who are recommended by their peers, and who don't have any
significant disciplinary or licensure problems. Although there is
a chance that a bad doctor may slip past their radar, this process
replicates, on a large scale, the kind of search you might do on
your own if you had the time and resources to do so. They offer
two levels of help: "*Best DocFinder*" is an Internet tool that allows
consumers to choose two referrals after searching by specialty
within a specific geographic region for $25; "*AcuMatch*" hooks
the patient up with a medical case manager who will do a personal search, and return three referrals. AcuMatch costs $975,
so it is best reserved for very complex or serious conditions that
require highly specialized care. Best Doctors can be found on
the Internet at www.bestdoctors.com, or you can call them at
1-888-DOCTORS (1-888-362-8677).

STEP 3: TALK WITH OFFICE STAFF

Once you've narrowed down your search, call the doctor's
office and ask to speak with the office manager. (Make an
appointment to call back if the manager is busy.) Find out the
nut and bolts of the doctor's business:

- Confirm that the doctor takes your insurance.
- Confirm the hospitals the doctor is affiliated with.
- Ask what the office hours and days of operation are.
- Ask how the doctor is contacted after hours or in case of
  emergency.
- Ask how long it takes to get an appointment for a regular
  physical, and for a patient with an acute illness.
- Ask if the doctor is usually on time for appointments, or if
  you should count on a wait. (Although waiting for an
  appointment isn't necessarily bad, since it may be a sign that

the doctor spends extra time with his or her patients, the office manager's answer will sometimes give you an inkling of any office-related problems.)

If the staff seems helpful and positive, and if you get the feeling that your needs would be met, ask to set up an appointment to speak with the doctor *in his or her office* to talk about the possibility of being treated there. Make sure the staff understands that you don't want to be examined (unless you do, in which case go ahead and make a regular appointment). At this time, ask if there will be a charge for speaking with the doctor. Many doctors don't charge for this kind of fact-finding visit, but some might. (If you make an appointment for an examination or second opinion, expect to be charged.)

If, on the other hand, the staff bad-mouths the doctor, treats you rudely, or gives you the impression that the office is in disorder, look elsewhere. A disgruntled staff is often a sign of office dysfunction, and you don't need to place your health in that kind of turmoil.

STEP 4: TALK WITH DOCTORS

When you've narrowed your list down to a handful of doctors, visit them in their offices to talk about the kind of care you want and to get a feel for the kind of care they might give you. Now is the time to talk about your desire to form a doctor-patient partnership and to participate in your medical care (as discussed in chapter 2). "Bring up that question directly with the provider," says Forrest Lang, M.D., of East Tennessee State University, an instructor on doctor-patient partnerships. "See what they say is their philosophical principle, and how do they respond to a question like that. If you don't like the answer, go find somebody else." Ask any other questions that might be important to you, including how the doctor views alternative/ complementary therapies, if the doctor takes e-mail questions from patients, if he or she will look at scientific studies you bring to appointments. Let the doctor know any special concerns you have for your treatment. Listen to the answers, but also to how the doctor answers. The doctor should listen closely to your questions, treat you with respect, make eye contact, take time to answer all your questions, and make you feel like a partner. Watch out for doctors who talk only in difficult-to-understand medical jargon. Good doctors should be able to explain things in everyday language.

If you are looking for a specialist, ask the tough questions related to experience: How many patients with your condition has he or she treated? How many died? What percentage survived long term? What are the usual outcomes? The more experience your doctor has, and the higher the survival rate, the better your chances of a good experience with that doctor. For example, one study by researchers at Johns Hopkins found that 98 percent of patients who had their prostate removed by highly experienced surgeons had no problems with urinary incontinence one year later, compared with a general average of 50 percent for all surgeons. On the flip side, watch out for extravagant numbers or tales of miraculous cures. In a less-than-qualified doctor, these claims may be inflated to get you to sign on as a patient. If numbers seem too good to be true, ask other doctors in the same hospital complex why they think that physician's outcomes are so good.

Ask a probing question or two about your disease or treatment. For example, ask what the physician thinks is the most promising recent development. This will allow you to judge not only how well the doctor keeps up with current literature but also whether he or she is willing to take a little time to educate you.

Ask the physician how he or she might coordinate care with any other physicians you may be seeing. You want a physician who is willing to write letters or forward medical records regularly to other physicians involved in your treatment, especially if those physicians don't typically interact. For example, a person with diabetes might be treated simultaneously by a PCP, a neurologist (nerve specialist), a nephrologist (kidney specialist), a cardiologist (heart specialist), and an endocrinologist (hormone specialist). Each doctor should know about each facet of care. If the doctor you're interviewing sees no need to communicate with other physicians, find a different doctor.

If, after all these steps, you find more than one doctor who fits your needs, consider yourself lucky and make a choice based on whatever criteria you like. All things being equal, the doctor you choose should be the one you trust the most to help you make the big medical decisions, the one you feel most comfortable with, and the one who will make you feel like an active participant in your own health care.

If you end up with no suitable doctors, consider relaxing some of the criteria in areas that should not affect performance. For example, if you've limited your search to only female physicians, repeat the process for male physicians, or expand your comfort zone of travel, or look at doctors affiliated with a different hospital.

Getting Second Opinions

The general motto after any diagnosis used to be "Get a second opinion." Although that advice is still sometimes important, it isn't as critical any more.

"There was a point in the past when there was so little information available to patients that to make sure you really had a good global feel for the disease you had to shop among several doctors to hear it presented to you in several ways," says Dr. William C. Dooley, of Johns Hopkins. "I believe we are beginning to get beyond that a little bit in that there's more and more information available. So that gradually over time as people begin to use Web technology, look for [information] more, they're going to be able to judge how correct the information is that they are being given."

If you have carefully chosen the doctors who treat you, done your own information searches, discussed what you found, and participated in making the medical decisions, a second opinion isn't absolutely necessary. There are times, however, when getting a second (or even a third) opinion from specialists makes sense. The following are some cases when you should search out a top-notch doctor or specialty medical center (see chapter 12):

- When your PCP diagnoses a serious or rare disease.
- When a diagnosis is uncertain or cannot be made.
- When current treatment isn't working.
- If surgery is recommended.
- If your doctor refuses to listen to your concerns or answer questions about treatment alternatives.
- If the doctor tells you there is no hope and refuses all further treatment. (In that case, find a new doctor. Even in advanced terminal conditions, doctors can participate by making patients comfortable in their final days.)

12. Hospitals

MOST often, the hospital you go to will be determined by the doctor you choose. If hospitalization is required, your doctor can send you to only one of the hospitals for which he or she has admitting privileges. Assuming that you've done your homework and have carefully chosen the doctor (see chapter 11), 90 percent of the time you won't need to do any additional work to find a good hospital.

But it's that remaining 10 percent that's tricky.

Most hospitals provide good basic care. The Joint Commission on Accreditation of Healthcare Organizations (JCAHO) rates and accredits hospitals across the United States based on a number of different factors. More than 97 percent of the hospitals they inspect meet the requirements to be considered generally accredited.

But if you have been diagnosed with a rare or potentially life-threatening disease, or if you are facing delicate surgery, you need above-average care. Depending on your individual situation, the relationship you have with your current doctors, and your health insurance, you may want to search out a hospital that offers you the best chance of survival and continued quality of life. Finding "the best" may mean traveling to another city or state, but many patients feel that the higher quality of care and better odds are worth the added inconvenience.

"Patients and their families need to make that initial decision of . . . how serious do I think my illness is and how far am I willing to go for its treatment," says Lillie Shockney, R.N., B.S., M.A.S., director of education and outreach at the Johns Hopkins Breast Center in Baltimore, Maryland. "If you have an ingrown toenail, you're probably willing to go four miles. But if you have cancer, you're probably willing to go a thousand miles."

This raises two main questions: (1) How do you know when the disease is serious enough to look for care outside your immediate surroundings? And, (2) How do you know which hospital to choose?

How Serious Is "Serious"?

There is no clear dividing line for when a patient should seek "outside" care. Several factors come into play:

The severity of potential outcomes of surgery: Every form of surgery carries risks, such as bleeding or infection. But some surgeries are relatively common and "easy," while others carry a relatively greater risk of complications. Talk with your doctor to get an idea of how complex and risky your surgery is. The riskier the surgery, the more likely it is that there will be quality differences among even specialty surgeons, and among the hospitals in which those surgeries are performed. "If you need your carpal tunnel problem fixed surgically, it may be that it doesn't make any difference whether it's fixed at the local hospital or if it's fixed elsewhere. But if you need an eight-hour high-risk operation to surgically remove your pancreas for pancreatic cancer, then it does make a huge difference," says John D. Birkmeyer, M.D., assistant professor of surgery at Dartmouth Medical School in New Hampshire. Anyone facing high-risk surgery should get a second opinion and investigate the quality of the surgeon and hospital.

The seriousness of the disease: The more life-threatening, disabling, or rare the disease, the better the chances that you'll need top-quality care. Some hospitals are simply better than others at treating specific diseases because they've had more practice at it, or because they are more technologically advanced.

Complexity of care: If you have a throat infection, any doctor can prescribe an antibiotic that will get the infection under control within days. But if your disorder requires an intricate balance of medications, careful monitoring, or continual evaluations and updates, consider going to a center that will provide you with the best training and information, and that will be most knowledgeable about advances (see Specialty Care Centers on page 205).

Time to consider: Emergency conditions don't allow the luxury of reviewing options or the physical ability to travel. For example, if you've got a perforated ulcer, you don't want to be getting on an airplane to fly halfway across the country for treatment. Similarly, research has shown that heart attack patients do just as well if treated in the closest hospital than if treated in a larger, more well equipped hospital. In emergencies, your best bet is to go to the nearest hospital.

Even if you determine that your disease is serious enough to warrant seeking treatment at an outside hospital, that doesn't mean that traveling is right for you. Medical care is a very personal decision, and an individual's feelings and beliefs play as much a part as objective numbers. Many people feel that traveling hundreds or thousands of miles away to be treated at a top medical center is not worth the trip. For them, being close to family and friends who can visit them in the hospital may be a more important consideration; or their trust in their primary care physician is so great that they cannot imagine being treated elsewhere.

"The downsides of excessive travel for a specific operation are not only inconveniences," says Dr. Birkmeyer, "but some of the continuity of care issues that occur when you physically separate where you live and where you get surgery." Surgery isn't necessarily a one-shot treatment, since complications can occur and follow-up visits are common. While some hospitals can coordinate follow-up care with the patient's hometown hospital, direct and easy access to the surgeon can be an important part of recovery.

These are valid points. In fact, they may be critical points. Research has shown that for some people, having the support of friends and family in a time of medical crisis can help the healing process. Ideally, each patient's decision will come after discussing options with physicians and specialists, and then carefully weighing the risks and benefits of outside care, the dangers and seriousness of the disease, the qualifications of the local hospital, and the patient's own personal preferences.

Of course, insurance coverage is also an important consideration. Every insurance plan is different. Some pay for everything and allow the patient to choose where they would like to be treated. Others may require a specific percentage of "out of network" doctor fees to be paid by the patient, while still others will cover only specific treatments in specific hospitals. Check with your insurance company to determine the scope of coverage before deciding where and how to be treated. (If, after reading the rest of this chapter and discussing treatment options with your doctor, you strongly feel that your best chances for survival are with a doctor or hospital not covered by your insurance, don't give up the fight. Ask your doctor and the hospital of your choice for options on how to get treatment there—some facilities have financial aid that allows them to treat uninsured or underinsured patients, and some may have a "plan of attack" that they've used to get insurance to cover other patients in the past. Talk to the physician gatekeepers at the insurance company to try to convince them that your life is at stake. Be prepared to present evidence of the higher quality of care at the hospital of your choice, including mortality statistics and other outcome measures. Ask your doctors to go to bat for you—for obvious cases, doctors often write letters or call the insurance company directly to plead your case. If all else fails, hire a lawyer to write a letter that again outlines the reasons for your need/desire to be treated at the hospital of your choice, and the ramifications to the insurance company if the lesser care they say they will cover results in a less-than-satisfactory outcome.)

Choosing a Hospital

HOSPITAL FACTS

If your doctor is affiliated with more than one hospital, or if you live near several hospitals and want to choose a doctor from one in particular, or if you are looking for a second opinion, or if your condition is serious enough to warrant looking for a more distant hospital that specializes in the treatment of your illness, you're going to have to do a little homework to find the right hospital.

There has been a lot of research in the past few years trying to determine what makes one hospital better or worse than another for treating specific illnesses, and there have been some interesting results:

Treatment varies depending on where you live: This phenomenon is called "regionality." For example, certain states have higher rates of certain procedures being performed than other states. One study conducted by researchers at the University of Minnesota in Minneapolis found that breast-conserving therapies (such as lumpectomy with radiation) were more likely to occur in San Francisco and Connecticut, and least likely to occur in Iowa and Utah (where mastectomy was more likely). Similarly, a Canadian study found that within the province of Ontario alone, rates of hysterectomy in one area were eighteen times higher than that of another area—for the same set of symptoms. Although some of this variation may be due to regional patient preferences, researchers feel that physicians tend to push the treatments they are most comfortable with, without necessarily considering the specific needs of individual patients. *Lesson: If you want or need a second opinion, look for one outside your immediate region to reduce the chances that both opinions will be the same simply because of regionality.*

Assembly-line surgery can be a good thing: Research has shown time and again that for certain intricate surgeries, high-volume hospitals have the best outcomes. Simply put, practice makes perfect. The more surgeries a hospital performs per year, the lower the death rates from those conditions, and the lower the rates of complications (see "High-Volume Surgery," page 209). One study published in the *Journal of the National Cancer Institute* found that men who underwent prostate cancer surgery at a low-volume hospital were about 50 percent more likely to die and 43 percent more likely to have a serious complication than those treated at a high-volume hospital (here, high-volume hospitals were those that performed more than 140 prostate surgeries per year). In these situations, it is the hospital—and not the doctor—that is the most important variable for recovery. In general, getting the worst doctor at a high-volume hospital is better than the best doctor at a low-volume hospital. But this doesn't mean that you have to go to one of the famous hospitals; most high-volume centers perform equally well. In fact, your local hospital may indeed be a high-volume hospital. *Lesson: For surgeries where high volume has been shown to be important, choose a hospital that does MANY. In some cases, a high-volume hospital may be within a twenty-five-mile radius of a low-volume hospital.*

Teaching hospitals tend to do better: Teaching hospitals—those affiliated with a medical school—treat rare, serious, and some not-so-serious conditions better than nonteaching or community hospitals. For example, research has shown that for some illnesses teaching hospitals have lower mortality rates than community hospitals. Why? Teaching hospitals tend to have more advanced technology. And because highly skilled specialists train students as well as treat patients, students and physician professors alike need to keep sharp and informed about the most recent advancements. *Lesson: Locate the nearest medical school and find out what hospitals they are affiliated with. Put them at the top of your list when searching for a good hospital.*

FINDING A HOSPITAL

Once you've decided that you want to find a good hospital, there are several steps you can take to ensure that you find one that will meet your needs.

Talk to your referring doctor or other trusted health professionals: It may sound obvious, but this is the most direct way to find a quality hospital, says Dr. John D. Birkmeyer. "Ask their opinion about the relative experience of the hospitals where [you] get most of [your] care, compared with other options in the region." Ask for advice throughout the process.

Call the nearest medical school: To find out which hospitals they are affiliated with, simply call the school.

Check MEDLINE: Refer to MEDLINE (see chapter 9) to find out which physicians might be among the top specialists for your disease, then call their offices to find out which hospitals they are affiliated with.

Check hospital "report cards": These shouldn't be used as the only criterion for judging a good hospital, but they can help point you in the right direction. The magazine *U.S. News & World Report* publishes an annual guide to the "Best Hospitals" by disease category. Although their rating process has been criticized for ranking such a small percentage of the country's hospitals on factors of questionable importance, the facilities that make the list are certainly among the best in the country. It's a helpful place to get an idea of where some of the top programs are located. (Ask the librarian in your local library to help you locate the most recent edition of that rating guide.)

Two websites that offer information about health care programs, surgical volume, and hospital "report cards" are Health Care Choices (http://healthcarechoices.org), a not-for-profit organization dedicated to educating the public about the health care system; and healthgrades.com (http://www.healthgrades.com), which offers health care report cards for hospitals, home health agencies, fertility clinics, nursing homes, and more.

Other report cards are more specific and therefore more helpful, but to a narrower band of patients. For example, some states (including New York and Pennsylvania) publish specific mortality information about hospitals and surgeons who perform coronary artery bypass surgery. Call your State Department of Health or health care council to find out what information is available in your state. Again, as tempting as it is to use report cards to judge the overall quality of a hospital, it's important to note that no report card tells the whole story.

"One thing they do," says Stephen T. Mennemeyer, Ph.D., associate professor in the School of Public Health at the University of Alabama, Birmingham, "is serve as a piece of information to consumers just so they can ask [additional] questions of their doctor or surgeon." If you read a disturbing report about your chosen hospital, talk with your doctor about it. There may be some special circumstances that have created what looks like a problem on paper, but which in fact turns out not to be a problem at all. For example, a hospital with a high mortality rate may simply admit sicker patients—or they may indeed be a bad hospital. Ask your doctor for details.

Check with specialty associations: Call or look on the Internet site for one of the organizations or associations that specializes in your disease—such as the American Diabetes Association, the American Cancer Society, or the National Multiple Sclerosis Society—to find listings of hospitals or treatment centers that specialize in those diseases (see "Specialty Care Centers," page 205).

Once you have a list of potential hospitals, work with your doctor to narrow them down to the best two or three options. Some important initial considerations might be whether your doctor is affiliated with that hospital, whether your insurance will cover the cost of treatment at that hospital, and how far you are willing to travel. Then, check out each hospital on your list a little further.

First, check to see whether your surgery is on the "high volume" list—that is, if volume has been demonstrated to be important to outcomes for your surgery (see "High-Volume Surgeries," page 209). If so, it is critical to seek out a high-volume hospital to lower your risk of death. How do you find out about volume? "Unfortunately . . . a patient can't just call up a hospital and say, 'Could you transfer me to the volume department,'" says Dr. John D. Birkmeyer. "Call up the surgeon's office and ask either the secretary of the surgeon or the surgeon to provide you answers to two questions: first, how many, on average, of these operations are done at this hospital, and second, how many, on average, of these operations do you do as a surgeon."

Next, find out about complication and mortality rates for your surgery or disease. Obviously, you'll want to go to a hospital that has the best track record for treating your type of illness. Look on the hospital's website for this information, or talk to the doctor or surgeon. If you can't get a straight answer, find another doctor or hospital. According to Lillie Shockney of the Johns Hopkins Breast Center, not freely giving this information tells you two unpleasant things: "Either they aren't monitoring themselves to know how they're doing, which would make me nervous to take my body there, or . . . they are hiding something, and that tells me I don't want to be part of their bad statistics."

Third, check to make sure that the hospital has been accredited by the JCAHO. You can do this either by visiting the website (www.jcaho.org) or by calling 630-792-5800. The JCAHO surveys and inspects about 80 percent of the hospitals in the United States. This is a voluntary procedure that can be considered a symbol of quality in itself. The hospitals that participate have a dedication to continued quality and quality improvement. At the JCAHO website, click on "Quality Check" to search by hospital name or geographic area for specific institutions. You can also see how that hospital was rated on all the evaluation factors on a scale of 1 to 5 (1 being the highest score, 5 the lowest). Once the basic information for the hospital you are searching for comes on the screen, scroll to the bottom and click on "View Performance Report." At the next screen, you'll notice more general information, and a "Contents" bar down the left side of the screen. From that left sidebar, click on the performance report you're interested in (most often that will be "Hospital Services"). This next screen will give you an overview of the rating; by clicking on "Areas Surveyed and Resulting Scores" you'll be able to see specific scores. If you have any questions about what you see on the screen, call the customer service telephone line to ask for help.

Finally, evaluate how comprehensive and specific the treatment program offered is. Some hospitals coordinate all aspects of disease care, from diagnosis and surgery to psychological services and nutrition education. It's not only easier on patients, it's better for their health. Research conducted at the Mayo Clinic in Rochester, Minnesota, has shown that, at least for breast cancer patients, treatment at these "multidisciplinary" groups had higher levels of physical functioning and satisfaction with their care (see "A Multidisciplinary Center in Action," page 207).

Once you've evaluated these factors and eliminated unaccredited institutions, choose the hospital that fits most of your criteria, and the one that makes you feel that you will be well taken care of. If you keep your PCP informed and involved in the decision, you'll have a good health advocate in your corner when you need it most.

SPECIALTY CARE CENTERS

Another option is to continue to use your local hospital and local doctors as your "home base" of treatment but also to seek additional help or second opinions at a special multidisciplinary treatment center, which is available for many disorders. These programs are usually located within a hospital, but treatment at that hospital isn't always necessary. (You will still need to check with your insurance company to find out about coverage.) They are staffed by physicians, nurses, nutritionists, and other health experts who are specialists in treating one particular disease—it's all they do, and they are great at it. They know all about the latest medications or medical devices, clinical trials (see chapter 16), and recently published studies that regular PCPs might not yet know about simply because they don't deal with them often enough.

For example, Brigham and Women's Hospital and Massachusetts General Hospital are affiliated with a specialized Multiple Sclerosis Center. "What we do here at our center," says Michael J. Olek, D.O., multiple sclerosis specialist, clinical instructor at Harvard Medical School, and attending physician at both hospitals, "is we go through the options for the patients and direct them in their care." Dr. Olek and his colleagues don't manage individual patients, they orchestrate treatment. "We have patients from all over the world. We're where people are sent for second opinions or other treatment options, and then we send them back to their general neurologist or MS neurologist." Patients generally return once a year or so for follow-up, but the bulk of their care is conducted at home by their regular doctors.

Another example is the Clinical Diabetes Center at Montefiore Medical Center in New York. Primary care physicians and specialists can refer their newly diagnosed patients to the center for special training in diabetes management. "Primary care physicians really don't have the time or skills to teach the patient how to make the decisions that really help keep their numbers under control," says Sheryl Merkin, M.S., R.N., C.D.E., C.P.T., a diabetes clinical nurse specialist at the center. The program works with the patient to educate and inform, and then follows up with the PCP to ensure good care over the long run. "The whole diabetes team sits down—an endocrinologist, a nurse educator, a nutrition educator—and we write down recommendations for the PCP so that any high-risk areas can be attended to," says Ms. Merkin.

These kinds of programs provide full-spectrum care for the illness while allowing the PCP and the patient to become more informed and empowered to make appropriate medical decisions. Ask your PCP about specialty programs for your condition, or check the websites of disease associations for programs near you. If your doctor won't refer you to one of these programs, seek another opinion and consider changing doctors.

A MULTIDISCIPLINARY CENTER IN ACTION

The Johns Hopkins Breast Center has been considered one of the best examples of a multidisciplinary center. I asked Lillie Shockney, the director of education and outreach at the center, to walk me through what might be typical for a new patient to experience. Here is her perspective:

It starts with diagnosis. If you're coming in for a screening mammogram and you have no known problems, a radiologist reads that film while you're here. If we see something, we'll do the spot films, and if we see something on the spot films that needs to be biopsied, we'll do that, too. Immediately. That is a wonderful way to help to reduce fear because there's no waiting.

If you've already been diagnosed, you would call the general breast center number, and they would connect you to the oncology referral office. There are people in that office that are specific for breast, for colon, for lung, for liver, for brain. The intake person would say, "I'd be happy to help you . . . tell me your problem." You may be crying, or you may be pretty steady on the phone. But she would find out from you that you have been diagnosed with breast cancer, and then complete a detailed worksheet to find out how much is known about the breast cancer. From that information, she knows what treatment protocol is likely and which doctor to schedule. Then, because she electronically has all the doctors' appointment schedules, she will schedule an appointment for some time within the next forty-eight hours.

If the patient is tearful while on the phone with that referral coordinator, the patient is given my name and number. When she calls, I'll try to calm her down, and arrange for one of our breast cancer survivor volunteers to meet and be with the patient during her initial visit.

During that first visit, they are given lots of educational material, including several color pictures to show anatomy and basic clinical information about breast cancer and its treatment, a resource section about social work and what they offer, cancer counseling center, our cancer survivor volunteer program and the importance of taking advantage of it, financial assistance information, and number for a national office for cancer survivors that helps people who are having employment or insurance problems. There's even a special document for husbands.

They are walked through the different treatment paths by the doctor. Then the survivor volunteer shows the patient and the family a photo album of what the different surgeries look like. So they get to see all shapes and sizes, all ages and races of women who have had all possible variations of surgery. After the photo album has been reviewed, the physician will ask that the patient take forty-eight hours to think about the decision.

The day before the surgery, the patient is booked for what we call the dress rehearsal, to see what's involved and meet the nurses. We'll tell them: This is the bra you're going to wake up wearing, and this is the drain and the kind of fluids it will have and how it works and why it's important. We want to reduce patients' anxiety to as low as possible. The best way to do that is to know every single thing that's going to happen on the day of surgery.

We like to call the day of the surgery "transformation day"—the day they are transformed from breast cancer victims into breast cancer survivors. When she wakes up in recovery, her family is brought back to be with her to celebrate her survivorship. The survivor volunteer is also there. She calls the patient the night before, sits with the patient during pre-op, and she is the first person the patient sees in the recovery room. We don't want the patient traveling though this experience alone. After surgery, the patient may go home, or she may stay, depending on what type of surgery has been done and how she feels.

She gets pathology information usually four days after surgery. Most patients want to know over the phone—they don't want to come in, they are too anxious. So the surgeon tells them. When the patient comes in to get her drain removed, she'll get a copy of that pathology report. We're trying to make sure she gets well-engaged in her treatment. Based on that pathology report, we know what the next treatment steps need to be.

If it's chemotherapy, we have a chemo class that explains what will happen. Patients get to know the type of medicine they'll receive, what it will feel like, side effects, what it looks like—some chemo agents are red and resemble blood, and we don't want them to think they are getting a transfusion.

Simple things like that keep patients from worrying to death. Now we're adding new programs to teach patients exercises, how to cook and eat healthier, and stress management. We're always trying to find a way to help patients learn to live with their new selves.

High-volume surgeries

R. Adams Dudley, M.D., M.B.A., from the University of California, San Francisco, and his colleagues reviewed the results of more than seventy-two studies that looked at the effects of volume on outcomes. After analysis, they found that certain conditions/ procedures had a significantly greater survival rate when performed by high-volume hospitals. If you need any of these procedures, seek out a high-volume hospital—the higher the better. Avoid low-volume hospitals:

Condition/Procedure	Definition of Low Volume
Coronary artery bypass surgery	less than 500/yr
Lower extremity arterial bypass surgery	less than 50/yr
Heart transplantation	less than 9/yr
Pediatric cardiac surgery	less than 100/yr
Coronary angioplasty	less than 400/yr
Elective abdominal aortic aneurysm repair	less than 32/yr
Carotid endarterectomy	less than 101/yr
Cerebral aneurysm repair	less than 30/yr
Esophageal cancer surgery	less than 7/yr
Pancreatic cancer surgery	less than 7/yr
Care and treatment of HIV/AIDS	less than 100/yr
Prostate cancer surgery*	less than 141/yr*

Source: Dudley, R. A., et al. Selective Referral to High-Volume Hospitals: Estimating Potentially Avoidable Deaths. *JAMA*. March 1, 2000; 283 (9): 1159–1166.

*Yao, S., and G. Lu-Yao. Population-based study of relationships between hospital volume of prostatectomies, patient outcomes and length of hospital stay. *JNCI*, November 17, 1999; 91(22): 1950–1956.

13. Complementary Medicine or Self-Care

As you search for health information, you'll undoubtedly come across advertisements, stories, websites, books, and medical journal articles that talk about "alternative," "complementary," "holistic" (or "wholistic"), and "natural" medicine. These types of remedies have been around for hundreds, even thousands of years, and publicity about these non-mainstream medical treatments has increased in recent years. U.S. consumers spend billions of dollars annually on self-care products and services, including supplements, herbs, homeopathic medicines, acupuncture, and massage.

For many consumers, understanding and integrating complementary medicine into their care can be complex, confusing, and costly. The questions most people want answered are: Do complementary therapies work? Which are best? Are they safe? How do I choose the best provider?

There are so many different modalities (meaning the different types or philosophies of treatment) that there are no short answers to these questions. But there are certain facts about the industry as a whole, safety concerns, and areas that show promise that you need to be aware of before deciding to try any nonstandard treatments for your disorder.

The Basics

You can start eliminating confusion based on the words used to describe the field alone.

Alternative: This word suggests that the nonstandard or complementary treatment substitutes for standard scientific medical treatment. So start by knocking the word *alternative* right out of your medical vocabulary. Every physician and every well-meaning, conscientious complementary practitioner will tell you that all treatments should be done in conjunction with your usual medical treatment, and that you should inform your physician before starting *any* treatment. This includes taking vitamins or herbs, going for acupuncture or massage, drastically changing your diet . . . anything. **Anyone who urges you to abandon standard treatment, or suggests that standard, scientific medicine is bad, or claims that prescription medications or chemotherapy are poisons, or tries to convince you to distrust your doctor is not looking out for your health. Run—do not walk—away from this type of practitioner.**
Natural: As much as we would like to believe that everything natural is necessarily healthy, it's not true. Many scams are perpetuated based on the idea that natural must be better than man-made. Don't buy this argument. Yes, many natural things are good for you, but nature can also be dangerous. Many poisons come naturally from plants, and bacteria and viruses are part of the "natural" world. In high enough doses, some herbs can cause an erratic heartbeat and death, and natural estrogens may be just as likely to cause gynecologic cancers as artificial estrogens (the research hasn't been done yet, but the potential is there). "Natural" does not always mean "good."
Holistic: This implies that the entire person is being treated, and yet virtually no nonstandard treatment will help with all aspects of your body, mind, and soul. The idea of being part of a

"holistic" treatment is appealing because we all want to feel loved and cared for. It is difficult to be a patient; after enough treatment, it's easy to start to feel as though we are little more than a disease wrapped in flesh. Yes, it is important to take care of yourself, inside and out. But the nonstandard medical modalities really don't offer true whole healing. They may help ease tension, create optimism, and make you feel cared for, but standard scientific medicine should also be part of the "whole."

Complementary: This is the most widely accepted of all the terms currently being used, but it, too, is not without controversy. In theory, "complementary" allows for standard medical treatments to continue while other, nonmedical therapies are tried. Some physicians, however, feel that "self-care" is a better term, since a great majority of people who claim to practice "complementary medicine" have no medical training, leaving patients to seek out the therapies on their own with no professional guidance. This chapter will continue to use the terms *complementary* and *nonstandard* to refer to treatments patients use along with their standard medical treatment to try to ease tension, reduce anxiety, and help in healing.

Risks of Complementary Medicine

Some physicians and scientists believe that all complementary medicine is potentially dangerous on a number of different levels. Others feel that noninvasive modalities (where nothing is put into the body) such as meditation and exercise are perfectly fine but that any invasive treatment carries risks. Still others are firm believers in one modality or another. Because of these different beliefs, advice about complementary medicines from any person or group will be biased, depending on their experiences. Patients need to be savvy consumers and apply the same critical thinking and decision-making processes to complementary medicine as they do to standard medicine.

There is currently a tremendous push in the medical community to conduct appropriate scientific research on complementary therapies. Until the research is complete, there are some facts about complementary medicines that are critical to the decision of whether or not to use them:

DANGER—BUYER BEWARE

At the worst end of the spectrum, some treatments can cause death either directly or by interacting with another product or medication. For example, some herbs can act as a blood thinner, and if a patient is already on a blood thinner for heart disease or stroke prevention, the patient would be at risk for abnormal bleeding. Other herbs can cause atrial fibrillation and death if taken in high doses. Shark cartilage (often taken by people diagnosed with cancer) can cause hepatitis or an elevation in liver enzymes that may be harmful in themselves, or may result in standard medical treatment being stopped prematurely. A study reported in the *New England Journal of Medicine* found an association between one type of Chinese herb used for weight loss and kidney damage and cancer. Even something as simple as aromatherapy massage may be harmful—one researcher discovered that some aromatherapists were using potentially toxic plant extracts and essential oils in their massage routines.

"Sometimes people aren't aware of the risks," says William T. Jarvis, Ph.D., professor of public health and preventive medicine at Loma Linda University in California, and coauthor of the textbook *Consumer Health: A Guide to Intelligent Decisions*. "This is one of the problems. People who take coffee enemas aren't aware many times that there are risks associated with it. We've seen people's bowels perforated by inserting the enema tube, we've seen septicemia [a blood infection], and because of the amount and frequency of having that many enemas, we've seen people's electrolytes upset and they can die from potassium depletion."

Since most remedies have not been thoroughly tested, there is really no way of knowing whether every product is safe, or whether there are long-term or undiscovered side effects or interactions. For this reason, there can be risks associated with taking nearly any herb, tincture, tea, or supplement or using any modality that involves eating, drinking, inserting things into your body, or applying anything to your skin. It all depends on what sensitivities you have, what other drugs or treatments you might be receiving, and what dosage you take.

NO REGULATION

Prescription and over-the-counter medications are regulated and monitored for safety by the Food and Drug Administration (FDA). There are strict standards that require manufacturers prove, through extensive studies, that the drugs they sell are safe and effective. But herbal products and many dietary supplements are not regulated for quality. Studies have found that two different capsules from the same bottle may contain differing amounts of the active ingredient. Even physicians who want to prescribe herbs to their patients admit that the quality control and standardization of most herbal products is poor. Until these products are standardized and regulated, you can't be guaranteed that you're actually getting what the label says.

But even the labels may be misleading. Congress has given tremendous freedom to supplement manufacturers regarding what claims they can make for their products. Although manufacturers cannot make unproven claims about treating diseases, they can make unproven claims about improving "body structure or function," and treating "natural states" or life processes such as acne, graying hair, aging, and morning sickness.

STANDARDS—NONE OR FEW

Since it is impossible to set treatment standards without proper research, there are no standards or guidelines for practitioners to follow for a majority of complementary modalities. Similarly, most have no standards describing the training and knowledge necessary for becoming a practitioner. In many cases, this means that just about anyone can send money to an organization for a particular modality, claim to be a healer, and receive a "certificate" that is virtually meaningless. This doesn't mean that the practitioner is necessarily out to scam the consumer (although this certainly can happen), but that it is extremely difficult to tell a "good" practitioner from a "bad" one.

"It's difficult," admits Ethan Russo, M.D., board-certified child and adult neurologist, clinical assistant professor in the Department of Medicine at the University of Washington School of Medicine in Seattle. "In investigating someone's background, I think it's reasonable to call and ask their office what their qualifications are—for example, whether they have had any formal training in one of the herbal schools. There may be a confusing set of initials behind people's names, and it's important for [consumers] to find out what those mean, because this is an area where a lot of people have opinions, and it's just a matter of how educated they are."

But even if you find out that a practitioner went to a particular school, how do you know how good the school is? There's really no way for the average person to know when it comes to complementary medicine; right now you're pretty much flying blind.

EFFECTIVENESS

For the most part, complementary therapies are untested, or tested and shown to be ineffective, or tested and shown to be potentially harmful. When practitioners are asked for evidence of what their treatments can do, they often point to their patients' success stories—anecdotal evidence that could just as easily have happened by chance. Some practitioners claim wondrous cures, but they fall apart under scrutiny. The miracles don't hold up if you look too closely.

Studies of some modalities, particularly herbs, are beginning to be conducted, but the results aren't always what herbalists would hope. A study published in 1997 looked at the effects of the Chinese herb dong quai, which has long been touted to relieve hot flashes and other menopausal symptoms. In a fully randomized controlled study, researchers found that the herb did not control menopausal symptoms any better than a sugar pill did. Does that mean dong quai doesn't work? No, it's only one study. But neither does it support the use of dong quai so far.

On the other hand, a few studies have shown that St. John's wort does seem to be an effective treatment for mild or moderate depression, but other studies have found that it can interact with some medications, making the drugs less effective. More research is currently being done.

"I'm not the kind of doctor to say, 'You can't take this,'" says James M. Metz, M.D., assistant professor of radiation oncology at the University of Pennsylvania and associate editor of the cancer website OncoLink. "Some of these things may turn out to be good. We just don't know yet, and that's why they are considered unconventional. A lot of therapies we have today are based on plants—Taxol is from the yew tree—so I'm sure there's something to some of these things, but we just have to work that out. Some of these things are hoaxes, and sifting through can be difficult. It's going to take time."

Once all the scientific evidence of the efficacy and safety of herbs and other complementary treatments is gathered, guidelines and treatment standards can be put into place, and using those treatments will become safer.

EXPENSIVE

Some doctors report that patients will try anything for a cure, and spend upward of $200, $500, or even $1,000 each month on unproven, unregulated, unstandardized treatments.

POOR PERFORMERS AND SCAM ARTISTS

Complementary therapy practitioners have no system for reporting harmful outcomes or incompetent performance. And since there is no central organizing body or sanctioning association, there is no way for practitioners to police themselves. Unknowledgeable, incompetent, and unethical practitioners can continue to practice without retribution.

Scam artists and unscrupulous, greedy merchants take advantage of the atmosphere of trust. Complementary medicine practitioners are often believed to be warm, caring, and nurturing people. And many of them truly are. But this general feeling of trust and acceptance means that it is easy for unethical individuals to take advantage of patients. Unfortunately, this is not a rare occurrence.

"We did this thing with [a national TV news show] where we went through one of the 'Whole Life' expos, and there was a booth there for a guy from [Mexico]," says Dr. William T. Jarvis of Loma Linda University. "He had these women who were claiming that this guy had cured them of breast cancer. The follow-up revealed that they were flight attendants who never had any disease, but they would lay over in Los Angeles on weekends, and they got paid to go there and make these testimonials. They picked up a few hundred dollars for lying through their teeth. You say, what kind of a person would do that? Well, there are people who are sociopaths . . . they will lie. They have no conscience. It's just a lark to them."

Because of all these factors, some physicians caution against using any form of complementary medicine. "It's the difference between going for a swim in the backyard swimming pool and going out into the ocean and swimming with sharks," says Stephen Barrett, M.D., board chairman of Quackwatch, a website that educates consumers about dubious medical information (www.quackwatch.com). "You might have some fun once in a while in the ocean, and maybe shark bites are not that common . . . but would you be comfortable [with the risk]? I wouldn't."

Dr. Jarvis agrees. He is particularly disturbed by the liars and cheats and unethical vendors he's seen. "If you try to match your wits with these kinds of people, you're going to lose," he says.

Using Complementary Therapy

Once you understand the basic facts about complementary medicine, you're already a more savvy consumer. And once you know that there are people in the world who will take advantage of your trust, who will lie to win your confidence, then you're at least going into the conversation with your eyes open.

So, are there any "safe" complementary therapies?

Perhaps. Scientific research has shown that the mind inter-acts with the body in ways scientists still don't understand. Complementary therapies that involve meditation, positive self-talk, relaxation, guided imagery, and prayer—when used in con-junction with standard medicine—will certainly make you feel better by putting you in a more positive emotional state, and may have physiological effects that promote healing. Exercise and other breath and movement therapies, such as yoga, t'ai chi, and qi gong, may also help keep your body healthy in some of the same ways that exercise is beneficial for all people, healthy or unhealthy: by improving strength and flexibility, and by giv-ing you an emotional sense of well-being. Other noninvasive therapies that are creative and enjoyable may also help improve mood and create positive mind-body interactions. These may include art therapy, music therapy, dance therapy, writing (journaling), and humor (as in laughter-is-the-best-medicine). And when used simply as calming techniques, aromatherapy and massage can be soothing and emotionally uplifting.

"I think a lot of these [mind-body therapies] really help patients, and I encourage patients to do them," says Dr. James M. Metz of the University of Pennsylvania. "Guided imagery in particular is great for people who . . . are nervous about their radiation therapy by getting them to relax. . . . It doesn't hurt, and it gives patients control over their lives at a time when they feel they've lost control."

These types of complementary therapies, always done together with standard medicine, can be used safely—*as long as they don't undermine the rationality of your standard medical therapy.* There is a tendency for some patients to abandon med-ical treatment if they believe their complementary treatments are helping them. Dr. William T. Jarvis tells the story of a woman who was scheduled for surgery. A nurse administered a "spiritual treatment" and "unruffled" the woman's "energy field." After being declared spiritually healed, the patient got up and left the hospital without receiving surgery. She felt it was unnecessary to go through the risks of surgery, anesthesia, and disfigurement when her spiritual side was healed. That patient was never heard from again. If she had stayed, she would have received the benefits of both spiritual and physical healing.

If you decide to try a complementary therapy, you should follow a few general guidelines.

Include your physician in the decision, and maintain your doctor-patient partnership. This point cannot be stressed strongly enough. Inform your doctor every step of the way, and let him or her know every new thing you try, even if it is as simple as taking a vitamin pill. (Case in point: Research has shown that some antioxidant vitamins may interfere with some chemotherapy treatments.)

Many patients are afraid to talk with their physician about complementary care. Dr. James M. Metz found that approximately 40 percent of the cancer patients in a study he conducted were using one or more unconventional therapies in addition to their standard medical treatment, but only 7 percent readily admitted to it in their initial meeting with the doctor.

"There used to be this don't-ask-don't-tell atmosphere [about complementary medicine]," says Dr. Metz. "Now, if you ask, they'll tell. People are beginning to feel a little more comfortable, and you just need to open the door for them a little bit . . . to make them feel comfortable enough to talk about it." By talking with the physician openly, patients have the opportunity to avoid dangerous drug interactions, or the chance that the complementary therapy will interfere with standard treatments.

In fact, physicians understand that many patients hear about and are considering complementary therapies. "For the most part, I think that they are OK," says Michael J. Olek, D.O., clinical instructor at Harvard Medical School and multiple sclerosis specialist. "I do ask patients to let me know what they are [using], and if I feel that they are harmful to the patient, then I'll say no. I don't think they have a benefit. However, [they do seem to give] a positive attitude to the patient."

And don't be surprised if your doctor brings up the issue before you do. "I encourage doctors, when they first diagnose a patient with a serious disease, to immediately open up the topic of unproven methods, alternative medicine," says Dr. William T. Jarvis. "They're going to read about it, they're going to hear about it from the media and their friends . . . so anytime a question comes up, invite [the patient] to talk about it. If the physician never heard about it . . . the patient can become the resource for more information."

A simple statement may be all that is needed to open the conversation, such as: "Doctor, I've heard about people with my condition who use a particular complementary treatment, and I've been thinking about trying it, too. Can we talk about how it might affect my medical treatment?"

Don't allow yourself to be flim-flammed. Watch out for the various tricks, rationale, and misleading advertisements that some practitioners use. Be wary of claims such as "no side effects," "we care about you," "our treatment attacks the cause of the disease," or "we offer an alternative." They may or may not be true, but they have nothing to do with healing.

Never allow a complementary practitioner without a medical degree to diagnose you, or to tell you that your physician has misdiagnosed you. If that happens, walk out the door.

If you want to try one of the noninvasive, safer treatments, learn the techniques in the simplest way possible. These are not difficult to learn, and many wonderful books have been written about meditation, relaxation techniques, and how to incorporate humor into your life. If you need to learn a skill, such as yoga or t'ai chi, find the least expensive teacher with the most experience in your area. You don't need to go to a high-priced spa or take years of lessons to learn the basics and use them for relaxation.

If you want to try one of the invasive modalities (such as herbs, acupuncture, or Chinese medicine), look for an M.D. who has taken additional training in that modality. Make sure the practitioner is willing to work with your current primary care physician.

Do your own research. You've done the research on your disease, now use the same techniques to research the modality.

Learn all you can. Read the positive and the negative aspects, and look for evidence for and against it so that you can come to an informed decision. "I use MEDLINE on PubMed," says Dr. Ethan Russo. "The intelligent, concerned consumer is going to be able to use this information to their advantage. They can call up articles and show their doctor what they found. . . . [But] I would be leery of commercial sites. If somebody is on the Internet and they see page after page after page of testimonials to ingredient X, but with no medical references to back it up, I'd be very suspicious." (See chapter 8 for a discussion on how to evaluate Internet information.) Also, choose high-quality books written by reputable authors (see chapter 5 for more information).

Carefully consider the information you find during your research. Don't jump at a new treatment that initially sounds good. If you decide to try it, and your doctor agrees, follow instructions carefully. For example, if you read that an herbal remedy was shown in a scientific study to be helpful for your problem, Dr. Ethan Russo recommends that you buy a product that uses the same standardized extract that was used in the study. This will require more research, since most herbal products in the average health food store are not standardized extracts. You'll have to refer back to the original study, then seek out an M.D. who has training with herbs to point you in the right direction.

Keep a record in your Personal Health Log of any complementary therapy you try. Note what you've tried, who the practitioner was, how the procedure was done, and how you felt, including any side effects. Keep a sample of any herb, vitamin, or supplement you take—put it in a plastic bag with a note describing what it is, when it was taken, and in what dosage and staple it to a page in your log. If you have any health problems because of the treatment, this record and sample will allow your physician to treat you effectively.

Perhaps in the future complementary treatments will be a part of proven and regulated aspects of all managed health care. Until then, tread carefully in this arena, and be honest with your physician about whatever you may be using.

14. Other Caregivers

IN the course of caring for your illness, you are likely to need or want the care and advice of a number of different types of health practitioners beyond physicians and specialists. The most common will be: pharmacists, dentists, physical therapists, dietitians, psychologists and psychiatrists, and support groups.

These experts act as part of your health team and should be used in conjunction with your primary care physician, not as substitutes for primary medical care. They perform functions that physicians either don't have time to do or for which physicians have not been trained. For example, in the Cleveland Clinic cardiology group, patients are treated not only by cardiologists but also by dedicated nonphysicians such as nurses, dietitians, psychologists, and physical therapists. "They actually spend a lot of time with the patients," says Gary Francis, M.D., director of the Coronary Intensive Care Unit at the Cleveland Clinic Foundation. "The problem in a busy clinic is, if I've got ten patients to see in a morning, there isn't time [for me] to counsel every patient." He and other physicians everywhere rely on qualified staff to handle different aspects of care.

For these adjunct experts, the criteria for choosing the best are the same criteria you would use to choose a good doctor: They should be professionally qualified and willing to form a health partnership with you. This means listening to your concerns, educating you about appropriate care and what your treatment options are, answering questions honestly and thoroughly, and being generally willing to help you through your illness within the bounds of their expertise. You should feel comfortable with them and able to trust their advice.

Your responsibilities, then, are also the same as what you would have with your primary care physician. That means being honest about your condition, even in embarrassing situations; asking questions if you don't understand what is being said; preparing for visits by writing down questions or concerns; and all the other activities you would do as an active patient seeing your primary physician. If at any time you feel uncomfortable with one of these health professionals, try to discuss the problem and work out a solution. If the professional is unresponsive, leave and find someone else to help you solve your problem.

Information is provided below for each of the major categories of health professionals, detailing what they do, when they might be necessary or helpful to your treatment, what qualifications to look for, and where to go for more information. (*Note:* If a particular health care expert is not listed here, search the Internet or ask your doctor for the name of a professional organization that certifies or trains that type of expert. Contact that organization to ask what specific qualifications you should look for.)

Pharmacists

WHAT THEY DO

Most people understand that pharmacists dispense prescription medications, but their true role as part of a patient's health care team is potentially much larger than that. Pharmacists are increasingly called on to help design therapeutic plans, monitor patients for side effects and drug toxicities, and ensure that the medications are actually doing what they were prescribed to do. A good pharmacist will contact other members of your health care team to consult or ask questions if necessary. "A lot of time, we suggest changes in medications," says Elaena Quattrocchi, B.S., Pharm.D., FASHP, associate professor of pharmacy practice at Arnold and Marie Schwartz College of Pharmacy in Brooklyn, New York. "We recommend certain changes, such as changing dosages depending on the patient's status, their age, and whether they have kidney or liver problems."

WHEN THEY MIGHT BE NEEDED

Everyone should have a good pharmacist, even if prescription medications are not required—pharmacists can also help guide choices of over-the-counter medications and supplements, and can provide expert information on how to manage certain health conditions (such as high blood pressure) to prevent future health problems. For patients who must take prescription medications, a good pharmacist can be one of your best defenses against drug toxicities or inappropriate medication. There are plenty of stories in the media of patients who have died or been harmed by having the wrong medication dispensed. No matter where the mistake originated, a good pharmacist with access to your health records would be able to catch the mistake in time to avoid problems.

WHAT TO LOOK FOR

1. A good pharmacist should be a willing partner in your health care, just like your doctor and other health specialists. Many of us have gotten so used to thinking of the pharmacist as the person behind the counter counting pills that we often forget that this is a trained health professional. Your pharmacist should be willing to come out from behind the counter, speak to you in confidence about your disorder and medications, and understand all your health needs. "You don't want to go to a place where they're not going to talk to you," says Dr. Quattrocchi. "You want to build up a relationship with your pharmacist . . .

you want the pharmacist to know you." Dr. Quattrocchi points out that daily stress, illnesses, diet, exercise habits, and even life changes such as a death in the family can affect the way medications work. You should be able to discuss these things with your pharmacist so that he or she can better monitor your health. (Once you find a good pharmacist, bring in your Personal Health Log so that he or she can fully understand your health needs.)

2. Along with personal conversation, the pharmacist should offer written information about the medications you'll be taking, including any potential side effects, when to contact the doctor, how long it will be until the medication starts to work, how and when to take the medication, and any recommended activity restrictions (such as "no driving" if the medication is likely to make you groggy or drowsy).

3. All pharmacists need to be licensed in the state in which they practice, and the license must be renewed every three years. Ask to see the pharmacist's license (which is usually hanging in the pharmacy) and check the expiration date.

4. Independent pharmacists generally offer more personalized care than pharmacists who work in chain drugstores, but this may be changing soon. Some chains, such as CVS and Eckert Drugs, are trying to improve the way their pharmacists interact with customers, and some are using mechanical devices to do the mundane pill-counting, leaving the pharmacist free to counsel patients. Interview pharmacists from several different stores and choose the one you feel most comfortable with. If they don't have time to talk to you, that probably isn't the pharmacy for you.

5. Some pharmacists attend certificate programs for certain diseases. Ask the pharmacist if he or she has attended any of these programs. "This is a clue that the pharmacy is very interested in patient care," says Dr. Quattrocchi. "They want to benefit their patients so they go through these programs so they know how to teach them." There are certificate programs for a number of disease states, including hypertension, diabetes, asthma, immunizations, anticoagulation, and AIDS. If you have

one of these disorders, you may want to choose a pharmacist who has had the extra training in your particular area. If you don't have one of these disorders, just knowing your pharmacist cares enough to go through the additional training could be an important consideration when making your choice.

6. The three big "don'ts" for choosing a pharmacy: *Don't* just go to the closest pharmacy. *Don't* choose a pharmacy based on price. *Don't* use more than one pharmacy. Choose a single pharmacy based on the quality of the pharmacist to ensure that your health is well looked after. "If you keep going to the same pharmacy, the pharmacist can make sure you're not duplicating medications and that you won't receive medications that interact with each other," says Dr. Quattrocchi.

7. If you find several good pharmacists in your area, some additional questions you may want to ask are:

- Do they have home delivery of medications?
- Can the pharmacist be reached by phone in case of questions or an emergency?
- What kinds of payments are accepted in the pharmacy? Do they accept HMO or third-party payments?
- Do they offer any special services, such as diabetes training, hypertension screening, bone-density screening, or vaccinations?

Note: Online pharmacies are generally not recommended because they are virtually anonymous pill-dispensers. They cannot offer the same full range of care that a local pharmacy can. If you must visit an online pharmacy, make sure:

- The pharmacy requires a prescription and works with your doctor. Do not allow an online doctor to diagnose or consult. And do not trust any pharmacy that does not require a valid prescription, since their overall quality controls are likely to be poor and could potentially jeopardize your health.
- The online pharmacy is licensed in your state.
- A pharmacist is available for questions, either by telephone or e-mail.

- The website is secure, with appropriate privacy and encryption measures in place.
- The site has received Verified Internet Pharmacy Practice Sites™ (VIPPS™) certification from the National Association of Boards of Pharmacy (NABP). This should be listed on the online pharmacy's website. A listing of all websites that meet the criteria for certification can be found on the website for the National Association of Boards of Pharmacy at http://www.nabp.net. (Click "VIPPS" on the selection bar, then on "List of Pharmacies.")
- Shipping and handling costs don't make the online pharmacy more expensive than your local pharmacy.

FOR INFORMATION

To find a good pharmacist in your area, ask your doctor, dentist, or other health professional for a recommendation. You can ask friends, too, but since so many people choose a pharmacy based on location, they may not be a reliable source of information about good pharmacists. Lists of local pharmacies can be found in the telephone book. If you have any questions about pharmacists and pharmacies, contact your State Pharmacy Association (listings for each state can be found on the Internet on the website for the National Community Pharmacists Association [NCPA] at http://www.ncpanet.org) or your State Board of Pharmacy (listings for each state can be found on the Internet at the website for the National Association of Boards of Pharmacy at http://www.nabp.net. Click on "Who We Are" and then on "Boards of Pharmacy").

Dentists

WHAT THEY DO

Dentists tend to tooth, gum, and mouth health. Although most people don't realize it, a qualified dentist should be an integral part of your health team. "There are many patients where we work hand-in-hand with their physician," says Richard H. Price, D.M.D., spokesperson for the American Dental Association, instructor at Boston University Dental School, and dentist in private practice in Newton, Massachusetts. "For example, the dentist can play a key role anytime there is reduced saliva flow. The side effect of two hundred to three hundred prescription medications is dry mouth—that includes antihistamines, antianxiety drugs, and cardiac medications. Saliva is your best natural defense against tooth decay and gum disease . . . so we work with the physician [giving patients] high-fluoride gels and [treatments to] supplement a dry mouth."

WHEN THEY MIGHT BE NEEDED

Every person should see their dentist at least twice a year for periodic cleaning and checkups. But if there has been a significant change in your medical condition, or if medications or treatments are affecting your saliva flow or mouth health, make an appointment to see your dentist more often. It is especially important for cancer patients to visit the dentist before beginning chemotherapy treatments, since chemotherapy drugs can cause mouth sores and may decrease general immunity. If you go into chemotherapy with a healthy mouth, there will be fewer chances for infection.

Cardiac patients may also want to see their dentist, since the buildup of plaque in the mouth has been associated with heart problems. "Did the heart problems cause bad gums, or did the bad gums contribute to the heart problems?" asks Dr. Price. "We don't know. But I know that it doesn't take much for bacteria to get into the bloodstream . . . and the bacteria that cause gum disease have the ability to cause clumping and stickiness." And stickiness in blood vessels may lead to atherosclerosis or blood clots.

Most important, don't skip or put off your regular dentist visit because you've been having other health problems—this may be exactly when you need your dentist the most. Your dentist is there to help you maintain good oral health throughout your illness.

WHAT TO LOOK FOR

1. A good dentist is part of your health team, a partner with both you and your primary care physician. One of the first things he or she should do is take a full medical history, as well as a dental history. In fact, it would be a good idea to bring a copy of your Personal Health Log to your dentist. At a minimum, you should provide your dentist with an updated list of your medications and physicians at each visit.

2. Check to see if your dentist is a member of the American Dental Association (ADA). Members are screened by the organization to ensure that they are fully qualified, licensed, and complete certain continuing education requirements. To find out if your dentist is a member, call the ADA at 312-440-2500, or visit the "Patients & Consumers" page of their website (www.ada.org), then click on "Find a Dentist: ADA Member Directory." *Note:* Not all qualified dentists are members of the ADA. If not, check to make sure your dentist meets requirements 3, 4, and 5 below.

3. A dentist should have a valid dental degree, either a D.M.D. (Doctor of Dental Medicine) or a D.D.S. (Doctor of Dental Surgery). There is no difference between these two degrees—different schools just choose to call the degree by different names.

4. Your dentist should have graduated from an accredited dental school. Ask your dentist from which dental school he or she graduated, then check with the ADA to see if the school is accredited (call, or look on the website at http://www.ada.org/prof/ed/programs/schools/us.asp).

5. Your dentist should also be licensed to practice in your state. Check with the American Association of Dental Examiners for the appropriate contact in your state (call them at 312-440-7464, or visit their website at http://www.aadexam.org).

6. Once you've established that the dentist is qualified and licensed, check the office. It should be clean and look professional. Safety issues are also important. Ask about sterilization procedures. All dental instruments should either be disposable (and disposed of after a single use) or heated to virus-killing

temperatures in an autoclave. If the dentist or staff is unwilling to discuss sterilization procedures, look for another dentist. Also, if you are not covered with a lead apron when X-rays are taken, walk out immediately and find another dentist.

7. The dentist should make you feel at ease. "The bottom line is personal contact," says Dr. Price. "Are you treated with respect? Are you treated as a person, not a walking tooth?" Talk with the dentist about procedures: What happens in case of an emergency? Are there alternatives to the procedures recommended? How much does the procedure cost? Will it hurt? According to Dr. Price, every patient walks into the dental office looking for what he calls the three Cs: cost, comfort, and cosmetics. If your dentist isn't concerned about those things, find a new dentist.

FOR INFORMATION

To find a good dentist in your area, ask friends if they are happy with their dentist or talk with other health professionals, such as your physician or pharmacist. Lists of local dentists can be taken from your area telephone book or from the ADA. No matter how you get the name, take time to meet the dentist, see the office, and evaluate the personality match before allowing any work to be done. In general, the best place to find information about dentists and dentistry is the ADA. They can be reached by phone at 312-440-2500 or on the Internet at www.ada.org.

Physical Therapists

WHAT THEY DO

"Physical therapists are primarily recognized as being musculoskeletal specialists, movement specialists," says Barbara Sanders, Ph.D., P.T., S.C.S., chair of the Department of Physical Therapy at Southwest Texas State University in San Marcos. They evaluate and treat people who have difficulty moving due to illness or injury. For example, a physical therapist is needed to help patients regain strength and proper movement after a broken bone has healed, or after a stroke or other debilitating event, or after hip or knee replacement, mastectomy, or other surgery that affects major muscle groups. Treatments generally include special therapeutic exercises.

WHEN THEY MIGHT BE NEEDED

Patients are referred to physical therapists by primary care physicians or specialists whenever disease or injury affects joint motion, muscle strength, or the ability to function in daily life. In some states, physician referral is required; in nearly all states, insurance will not cover nonreferred patients.

WHAT TO LOOK FOR

Most important, you want to be sure that the physical therapist is licensed—and all states require licensing. You can find out if a particular physical therapist is licensed by calling your State Board of Physical Therapy. The phone number and address of your state's board can be found by contacting the Federation of State Boards of Physical Therapy (on the Internet, go to www.fsbpt.org, then click on "Directory of State Boards," or call at 1-800-881-1430).

Then, just as with physicians and hospitals, find out if the therapist or therapy group handles your type of problem often. Ask how many patients with your problem they've helped in the past year; then, if you have a choice of centers, go to the one that has handled the most cases similar to yours.

There is also a partnership component to working with physical therapists. "Look for someone who will thoroughly explain the treatment—what will happen, the positive, the negative—then decide if you choose to participate," says Dr. Sanders. Once the therapist takes the time to explain what's going on, you should work together to establish goals. Then the therapist can determine how many treatments it will take. The therapist should also take the time to explain the kind of physical demands that will be placed on you. "There are some treatments that will cause pain—that's just the way it is. But it shouldn't be excruciatingly painful, and the therapist should take that into consideration and never push patients beyond their pain tolerance." By working together in partnership, you can reach your goals in the quickest way possible for you.

There are a few specialist physical therapists who may be better trained to take care of your problem. The specialty areas are pediatrics (specializing in treating children), geriatrics (specializing in treating older people), sports, cardiopulmonary (dealing with heart and breathing difficulties), neurology (dealing with brain and nerve dysfunction), orthopedics (dealing with issues of movement and daily function, exercise physiology and biomechanics), and clinical electrophysiology (use of electrical testing and nerve stimulation). The main difficulty with choosing a specialist is that there are so few of them, so it may be difficult to locate one in your area.

FOR INFORMATION

Ask your primary care physician, other health professionals, friends, and family for recommended physical therapists. You can also call the state chapter of the American Physical Therapy Association (APTA) to ask for names of therapists in your area, or with a particular specialty. You can find the state chapter's phone number or website from the APTA (on the Internet, go to http://www.apta.org/Components/component_home_pages, and where it says "Chapters" click on the pull-down arrow to find your state, then click on "Go," or call at 1-800-999-2782).

Dietitians

WHAT THEY DO

Dietitians are trained in all aspects of food and nutrition. They conduct a thorough analysis of each patient, including medical history and current diet, and advise the patient on how to control the disease through diet or how to overcome eating difficulties caused by the disease while still maintaining a healthful diet.

WHEN THEY MIGHT BE NEEDED

Dietitians are involved in wellness and disease prevention, as well as in treatment. After a diagnosis, dietitians are most helpful for illnesses related to digestion or metabolism (such as Crohn's disease, diabetes, or celiac disease), or if the illness or its treatment causes changes in weight or the ability to eat (such as with cancer, eating disorders, or autoimmune disorders). Anyone who wants to learn to eat a more healthful diet can see a dietitian, but most insurance companies will cover only illness-related dietitian referrals.

WHAT TO LOOK FOR

Not all states require or even have licensing for dietitians. If your state does, make sure the dietitian you visit has a license to practice in your state. (To find out if your state requires licensing, call your state's department of health or visit the regulations page of the American Dietetic Association website.) Many people who claim to be "nutrition consultants," "nutritionists," or "dietary specialists" haven't had appropriate training. Avoid any dietitian or nutritionist who is not an "R.D."—the initials that tell you that the person has gone through an extensive training and internship process to become a "Registered Dietitian."

FOR INFORMATION

Check with your hospital to find out if they have a licensed or registered dietitian on staff. You can also call or visit the website of the American Dietetic Association (1-800-366-1655, www.eatright.org) to find a registered dietitian near you.

Psychologists/Psychiatrists

WHAT THEY DO

Mental health professionals can help people deal with stress and trauma, including those brought on by illness. Psychologists and psychiatrists both may use a variety of techniques, including one-on-one counseling sessions, group therapy, family therapy, or behavioral therapy that works to change habitual patterns of reacting, such as learning new ways of coping with stress. In addition, psychiatrists can prescribe medications that may help patients out of their depression or relieve anxiety.

WHEN THEY MIGHT BE NEEDED

You should seriously consider consulting a mental health professional

- If you feel that your life is "out of control," or
- If you "can't cope," or
- If your emotions are causing you to sleep or eat more or less than usual, or
- If your work or home relationships are suffering, or
- If you need help finding ways of coping with and managing your disorder emotionally, or
- If you feel that life isn't worth living.

In addition, psychologists and psychiatrists can be specifically helpful for people with illnesses. Therapists are often used to help patients control high blood pressure, reduce headache frequency, control chemotherapy side effects, change health-harming habits, and manage chronic pain. And some studies have shown that patients who receive counseling before surgery have shorter hospital stays, need less pain medication, and have fewer complications. Ask your physician if there are any aspects of your disease that might be helped through counseling.

WHAT TO LOOK FOR

First, make sure the therapist has proper credentials. For a psychiatrist, this means having a valid M.D. license plus a specialty certification in psychiatry (see chapter 11). This means that psychiatrists not only graduate from medical school, which makes them qualified to prescribe medication, but they have had additional training in psychological practices. You can find certified psychiatrists online at the American Board of Medical Specialties website (www.certifieddoctor.org). For a psychologist, you'll want to find someone with a Ph.D. (Doctor of Philosophy) in clinical psychology, or a Psy.D. (Doctor of Psychology). Both types of degrees will ensure that the psychologist has had doctoral-level education and training.

Note: Although the Ph.D. and Psy.D. degrees are signs of extensive training, counselors may practice with a master's (M.A., M.S., or M.S.W.) degree. These professionals may work in private practice, community health centers, or government organizations. Licensing and certification standards vary from state to state. Check with your state's Board of Examiners for Psychology to find out requirements, then make sure your counselor is practicing legally. Word of mouth from friends and other health professionals is the best way to locate a good counselor.

Second, the psychologist should be licensed to practice in your state. All states require psychologists to be licensed. If the psychologist is a member of the American Psychological Association (APA), then he or she must be appropriately licensed and credentialed. But not all psychologists belong to the APA. To check on the licensure status of a non-APA psychologist, contact your state's Board of Psychological Examiners. You can find the phone number by calling your state's Department of Health, or by doing an Internet search.

FOR INFORMATION

Ask friends and health professionals if they have had any good experiences, and if they could recommend a psychologist or psychiatrist. For more information, or for a referral to a psychologist in your area, call the American Psychological Association (APA) at 1-800-964-2000. Be sure to tell the counselor why you are looking for a psychologist—some specialize in dealing with serious or chronic illnesses, so you'll want to get a referral to someone with as much experience in those areas as possible. The APA website also offers lots of other helpful information (www.apa.org). For referral to a psychiatrist, talk with your primary care physician. That referral will have to be treated as any other referral to a medical specialist.

Support Groups

WHAT THEY DO

Support groups can be useful in helping people deal with the stress of illness and other life crises. There are many different types of support groups. The most basic could be as simple as a few friends with the same illness getting together for coffee once a week to talk about their experiences. Most support groups, however, are started by hospitals or disease organizations. Although some are strictly composed of people who have a particular disorder, many have professional psychologists, nurses, or physicians who help guide the group.

It's important to understand that research into the value of support groups is ongoing. Although studies have documented that support groups can help provide relief, reassurance, hope, anxiety reduction, information, guidance, and emotional support, some may also cause additional stress or provide misleading or depressing information. In short, all support groups may not be right for everyone.

Studies by Vicki Helgeson, Ph.D., associate professor of psychology at Carnegie Mellon University in Pittsburgh, Pennsylvania, and her colleagues have shown that support groups that provide education as a key component were helpful for everyone, while groups that focused more on emotional support were helpful only if the patient did not already have a good support group in place, such as friends or a supportive spouse. In one study on the effects of different types of support groups for breast cancer patients, Dr. Helgeson and colleagues found that physical health actually decreased in women who had good outside support but attended an emotional-type support group, while women who had little or no outside support improved their physical health by going to the same group. The lesson: Not everyone benefits from all support groups. Don't allow yourself to be bullied into joining if you don't feel it is necessary, or if you don't feel the benefits once you have gone a few times.

Another debate has arisen over whether support groups can actually help prolong lives (as in the case of advanced cancer patients). A 1989 study conducted by Dr. David Spiegel from Stanford University found that women with metastatic breast cancer who attended support groups generally lived longer than those who did not attend support groups. His research has not been reliably replicated, which means that even if it is true, the effect is not strong or consistent. More recent research, notably by Dr. Alastair Cunningham of the Ontario Cancer Institute in Toronto, found no evidence of increased survival in women with metastatic breast cancer. More research is currently being done. The lesson, again, is not to be forced into a support group if it's not what you want.

One newer development is the formation of support groups on the Internet. "You might call this a support group without walls," says Maurie Markman, M.D., director of the Cleveland Clinic Taussig Cancer Center in Ohio. "You literally dial up online and find people with your disease, with similar experiences, with similar types of therapies. And just as we talk about support groups in cancer as very important to an individual because you can talk to someone who has . . . experienced it, gotten through it—something that a physician can never do unless he or she has actually gone through it—if you're on the line with the right people, you could potentially get some very valuable information." The potential downside, of course, is the same as with any unprofessional information found on the Internet: The information might be misleading or even dangerous. Many physicians recommend that if you use an Internet-based support group, look for one that is moderated by a professional, and don't use it as your sole source of information.

WHEN THEY MIGHT BE NEEDED

Support groups are helpful whenever a patient feels the need to talk with other people who have the same disorder. One study found that people tend to join support groups for diseases that carry a higher stigma (real or imagined), such as HIV/AIDS, breast and prostate cancer, as compared with diseases with no perceived stigma, such as heart disease. This is probably because patients feel less comfortable talking about their concerns with family and friends if it means talking about something potentially embarrassing. According to Linda Farris Kurtz, D.P.A., professor in the Department of Social Work at Eastern Michigan University, people who are extremely upset should wait until they are more emotionally stable before joining a group. "Groups are all so different," says Dr. Kurtz, "and while most group members respond positively, they may end up with a group that's quite large and they may not get the individual attention they need." This would mean that the patient would have a bad group experience, possibly feel worse, and perhaps not attend any other group meetings.

WHAT TO LOOK FOR

1. Look for a support group that has structure and provides education. "I would advise [someone] who was looking into a support group to talk to the person who's running the group, and find out what usually happens," says Dr. Helgeson. "If the person says that it's relatively unstructured, and people just kind of sit around and talk and share feelings, that would be a red flag that it might not be such a good group." But if the group leader can hand you a schedule of speakers that includes doctors, nurses, nutritionists, and other professionals, then it's a good sign that the group is dedicated to providing its members with as much information as possible.

2. The group should be welcoming. Watch out for groups that form cliques and don't warmly welcome new members. "That would be very unusual," says Dr. Kurtz, "because groups usually want newcomers more than anything. If you walk in and feel like you don't belong, that's a bad sign. Turn around and leave."

3. "Stay away from a group that's doing a lot of complaining

or emoting," says Dr. Kurtz. "Particularly about the medical system. That can be very discouraging to other people who are depending on the medical system for their care."

4. Look for groups that have members who are in a similar position—with a similar disease at a similar stage. It can be very discouraging for someone who is newly diagnosed to be exposed to people who are dying of the same disease. That dying person's disease path may not be the same as that of the newly diagnosed person.

5. The group facilitator shouldn't be doing all the talking. Group members and professional speakers should have a chance to talk. There are no specific qualifications necessary for a good group leader other than the ability to encourage discussion and organize informative meetings. Physicians, psychologists, social workers, and other patients can all be effective leaders.

6. Avoid groups that encourage members to express a lot of intense feelings. Yes, feelings will be expressed during a group, but people should not be expected to bare their emotional scars. After all, no one will be there to support the patient once they go home at the end of the group. "Emotional support is good when people are talking about their concerns and feelings," says Dr. Kurtz, "and the other members of the group can identify with that and talk about how they've gotten past it . . . you feel this way today, and I used to feel that way, but that feeling will go away. So it's about recognizing the feelings, but not forcing the person to experience or talk about them."

7. Unless the group is being run by a physician, avoid groups that give advice about medical therapies, treatments, or drugs. It's fine to talk about ways to combat certain side effects or to share personal experiences, but only a physician should provide medical advice.

8. Trust your instincts. Try a group. If you don't like it, don't go back. It's not considered rude, and it's better that you find a group you like than to stick with one you don't like out of a misplaced sense of obligation.

FOR INFORMATION

To find out about support groups in your area, ask your doctor or call your local hospital. Call or visit the website of a disease association (such as the American Cancer Society) for your disorder. On the Internet, go to the *healthfinder* site (www.health finder.gov) and type in "support groups" to find organizations and clearinghouses with support group information.

Putting It All Together

15. Understanding the Numbers

MANY people dislike dealing with numbers. We tend to avoid them in day-to-day life, and many of us have terrible memories of math in school: embarrassing trips to the blackboard to figure out a problem in front of other students, frightening standardized tests, and confusing "word problems" that always seemed to involve trains leaving the station at different times. If you broke out in a sweat just reading this paragraph, take a deep breath and relax. This won't be painful.

Why You Need to Understand Numbers

Anyone who reads or hears medical information will be confronted with numbers in one form or another. Doctors use numbers to communicate specific information about diseases and treatments in a way that is precise and strictly defined. Risks, benefits, chance of recovery, average recovery time, significance of study results, and treatment comparisons are often presented in terms of numbers. All scientific knowledge comes from research studies, and all research studies are interpreted through statistics (a fancy way of saying that the results are analyzed with numbers).

You don't have to be a mathematician to understand what numbers mean, but you may have to spend a little time getting used to this new language before you'll feel comfortable with it.

A Word About Research Studies

Numbers are precise, but they are only meaningful if they are interpreted correctly by the researchers who generate them. In particular, researchers must accept that all people are not the same, and those differences change the way people respond to medical treatments. Statistics are used to express the degree of confidence researchers have in their results. In other words, statistics are tools that allow researchers to estimate how much of the difference they observe is just because people are different, and how much is because they have figured out how to treat a disease. This can be mind-boggling for those of us who are comfortable with the certainty of "2 + 2 = 4."

Statistics are an important part of any scientific study because of variability. Different people respond differently to the same medical treatment, and measurements of the same quantity can change. Consider your weight as an example. Perhaps you have to work hard to lose even a pound, but a friend can lose several pounds in a week or two with the same exercise routine. Different people can have different changes of weight under the same conditions.

What's more, your own weight is fluctuating all the time. Anyone who has watched their weight knows that the scale will give different readings at different times of the day, depending on how much you have eaten, drunk, and perspired. After a sweaty exercise session, your weight might be more than a pound lighter, but after you have a glass of water or two, it goes right back up again.

This same variability, from person to person and from moment to moment, occurs in almost every medical measurement. Good medical studies are designed to allow doctors to observe the effect of the treatments being tested despite this inherent variability. Because of this, the results of these studies are not definitive but are instead stated in terms of a likelihood or probability.

For example, a study testing the effect of calcium supplements on blood pressure might conclude, "This study provides strong evidence that calcium supplements reduce seated systolic blood pressure in healthy black men between the ages of 25 and 45." In this conclusion we see the researchers needed to frame their results precisely; the kind of blood pressure reduced is described carefully, and the target population is delimited. But notice that the conclusion doesn't state that calcium supplements reduce blood pressure, just that there is strong evidence that this is so. Conscientious researchers realize that the natural variability of the subjects in their test might have combined in just the right way to give the results that they have observed. This would be a very unlikely coincidence, but we all know that unlikely coincidences do sometimes happen. So conscientious researchers don't make definitive statements when natural variability might be the explanation, no matter how unlikely that might be. Later in this chapter, in the section on "Significance, Probability, and Confidence," we will delve into how researchers communicate their degree of confidence in their results using statistics.

The way a study is designed, the kind of subjects included in the study, the way a treatment is administered, and uncontrolled outside influences (known in scientific circles as uncontrolled "variables") can all alter the kinds of numbers that result from scientific research. For example, if researchers want to compare two different kinds of treatments, first they need to define the target population narrowly (healthy black men between the ages of twenty-five and forty-five in the example above).

Then they must choose a pool of subjects from the population that is as representative of the target population as possible. Choosing subjects that have too much in common would limit the usefulness of the study. For instance, researchers try to assemble a pool that avoids containing many subjects who are blood relatives, or live in the same neighborhood, or work at the same place or in the same profession. Any thread of similarity among the subjects might bring the results of the study into question.

Finally, the researchers must make certain that the subjects in a study are assigned to treatments randomly. If Treatment A is tested only on men and Treatment B is tested only on women, the results cannot properly be compared because the groups used were so different. Men and women may respond entirely differently to the treatments. The findings would tell you absolutely nothing about how Treatment B would work on men (or, conversely, how Treatment A worked on women). Numbers would be generated, but they would be of little value in actually determining how well one treatment worked compared to the other. If subjects are chosen from the target population as a whole and assigned to treatments randomly, the variability of the entire population is spread out evenly, and neither treatment gets an unfair advantage.

Of course, good research studies strive to control as many different factors as possible so that the chances are greater that they get accurate, reliable, and meaningful information. The lesson for nonresearchers is that numbers are important, but they are only as valuable as the study design and the interpretation. (See chapters 6 and 9 for more information about types of studies and how to evaluate them.)

The rest of this chapter will describe some of the basic terms you may come across during your information search and in discussions with your physician. This list is not intended to be comprehensive; if you find a term not covered here, ask your doctor to explain it to you. Also, the definitions are intended to help you understand basic concepts—they won't necessarily meet a statistician's standards of precision. Anyone who feels the need to understand statistics in a more in-depth way can consult basic statistics books, such as *Introductory Medical Statistics* (third edition, by R. F. Mould, IOP Publishing, 1998) or *How to Think About Statistics* (by John L. Phillips, Jr., W. H. Freeman Publishers, 1999).

Example of a Simple Research Study

In order to illustrate the various concepts and terms defined below, let's set up a simple experiment: Imagine that you want to find out whether caffeine really does keep people awake. You invite thirty of your friends and colleagues to your house for a dinner party. They will act as the *subjects* (the people you will be testing) in your experiment. We expect that these people form a representative sample of the wider population of interest—say, healthy adult Americans. (This would not be true, however, if your friends all came from your sleep-disorder support group, for instance.)

For the purposes of our study, we will assume that on a typical evening all our subjects go to bed at midnight and fall asleep immediately, and that no one has a medical condition that will be made worse by drinking caffeine. In a real experiment, all these *extraneous variables* (outside factors that might affect the outcome of the study) would be controlled by narrowly defining the target population or controlling the subjects' surroundings during the study. Researchers are often able to apply statistical techniques to smooth out some of the unwanted variability in the data they collect to arrive at summary numbers nearly as simple as those we offer below.

We will test three different caffeine levels as our *independent variable* (the factor that we are manipulating in the experiment) by serving three different types of coffee after dinner: caffeine-free; regular caffeinated coffee; and double-strength coffee. For our *dependent variable* (the factor we will measure to see the outcome of the experiment), we will call everyone the next day and ask what time they fell asleep. (We are going to make a gross assumption that our subjects will know the time they fell asleep.)

It is important that the study includes decaffeinated coffee even though we are interested in studying the effects of caffeine. This is called the *control* treatment. It allows us to discount the effect of attending this particular dinner party on the times when people fell asleep.

Since we have thirty people coming over, and three different strengths of coffee, we'll assign ten subjects to each *condition* (the particular level or type of factor we are manipulating). You may see this written in medical journals as $n = 10$. The letter n means number of subjects.

Once all thirty people have arrived, we will *randomly assign* the subjects to each condition to ensure that the subjects in one condition are roughly equivalent to those in another condition. Each subject will close their eyes and choose a piece of paper from a hat that has a number on it: 1, 2, or 3—corresponding to the three different experimental conditions. They will be served coffee only from pots labeled with the same number. Each subject will be served three cups of coffee over the course of the evening, and we will assume that everyone finishes drinking all three cups. Ideally, we would have a neighbor come over before the party to put the different-strength coffees in the pots, leaving us a note to open in the morning telling us which number went with which strength. This way we cannot possibly let the guests know who is getting which treatment because we do not know ourselves. This is called a *double-blind* study since neither the subjects nor the researchers know what kind of treatment is being given to which subjects. Everyone goes home at 11 P.M., and it is assumed that they will all try to go to bed at their usual time of midnight.

The next day, we call and ask what number was on their paper (to know what type of coffee they drank) and what time they fell asleep. The time difference between midnight (the usual sleep time) and the time they report will be our measure of how much of an effect caffeine had on their sleep. For example, if someone reports that she did not fall asleep until 3 A.M., the difference between midnight and 3 A.M. is three hours. Since we've tried to keep everything else the same, we'll assume that those three hours of sleeplessness reflect the effects of caffeine.

The imaginary results for our experiment are as follows. Each number represents the number of hours until sleep for an individual subject:

Decaffeinated	Regular Caffeine	Double Caffeine
1	1	2
0	1	3
1	1	2
0	3	4
2	2	3
0	1	5
1	3	3
0	2	4
1	3	5
0	2	3

This is a small example of the type of *raw data* (unanalyzed numbers) with which scientists begin. In a real medical study, scientists might make several different measurements on thousands of subjects. Then, through statistical analysis, they try to make sense of what the numbers mean. We will refer back to this table to illustrate some of the more common statistical terms.

The Basics: Averages and Percentages

The easiest way to characterize information is to talk about averages and percentages. By *average*, we generally mean "typical," but there are three different ways to define an average:

MEAN

The mean is the sum of all the numbers for a given condition divided by the total number of subjects in that condition. For example, to get the mean for the double-caffeine condition, we add up the hours-till-sleep for all subjects in that condition and divide by 10 (the number of subjects).

$$2+3+2+4+3+5+3+4+5+3 \, /10 = 34/10 = 3.4$$

You'll notice that no one actually took 3.4 hours to fall asleep, but that is the mean average of how long it took that group. (If you want to try this for yourself, the mean for the decaffeinated group is 0.6, and the regular caffeine group is 1.9.) When you see the word *average*, you can usually assume that it is the *mean* unless otherwise specified.

MEDIAN

The median is the middle observation if all the observations are put in order from lowest to highest. If there are an even number of observations, as we have in our case with ten different subjects, choose the average of the middle two observations. For example, if you reorder our double-caffeine numbers by value, they look like this: 2, 2, 3, 3, 3, 3, 4, 4, 5, 5. The median would be the number between the fifth and sixth number. But since the fifth and sixth numbers here are both 3, the median is 3. Notice that this is a slightly different way of describing the average as compared with the mean, with a slightly different "average" number. (The median for the decaffeinated condition is 0.5, and regular caffeine is 2.) The median is less affected by isolated extreme observations than the mean. Suppose one of the subjects who reported taking five hours to fall asleep after having double-strength coffee called back and changed her answer. She actually didn't fall asleep until 9 A.M., nine hours after going to bed. This will increase the mean to these observations from 3.4 to 3.8, but it doesn't change the median at all. Beware of this difference when reading medical literature. If the author wishes to underplay the significance of a few extreme observations (also called *outliers*), the median will be used to summarize the results. If the author's point is better served by highlighting the effect of one or two extreme observations, the mean will be the summary offered. (Imagine if you found out that the "average" starting salary of anthropology majors in a particular year was $100,000. It might make you want to go back to school to study anthropology. But then imagine discovering that all but one of the newly graduated were making less than $30,000. The exception: Michael Jordan, the basketball superstar and anthropology major, whose enormous, nonanthropology-related salary gave misleading "average" results. The *mean* was $100,000, but the *median* would probably be around $19,000.)

MODE

To find the mode, look for the number that appears most often in the series. For example, in the decaffeinated condition, the number zero appears five times, which makes it the most common number, and therefore the mode. (The mode for the regular caffeine condition is 1, and double-caffeine is 3.) The mode is really useful only in studies where there are many observations. A real study with only ten subjects per treatment generally would not use a mode. The mode is like the median in that extreme observations don't affect it much.

Percentages are used to talk about a particular amount, fraction, or proportion in relation to the whole. One hundred percent means all, everyone, everything—the biggest part possible. Similarly, 50 percent is half and 25 percent is a quarter. For example, we can say 100 percent of the people who were our subjects in the caffeine experiment eventually fell asleep. That means *all* thirty subjects fell asleep sometime, no exceptions.

Any smaller percentage is found by dividing a particular amount by the total amount, then multiplying by 100. So if we wanted to find out what percentage of all our subjects took two hours or more to fall asleep, we would count the total number of twos, threes, fours, and fives, then divide that number by the total number of subjects (thirty subjects in all). In this case, seventeen people took two or more hours to fall asleep: 17/30 is .5667, multiplied by 100 is 56.67 percent. This means that slightly over half our subjects took more than two hours to fall asleep, and that makes sense since seventeen is just slightly more than fifteen, half of thirty.

In a medical environment, you may read that 70 percent of people who received a particular treatment had side effects, or that 1 percent of patients had to have a second surgery. You can use these numbers to gauge how likely it is that you might have a similar experience, based on what happened to others. Of course, every person is different and your response may not be the same as those of the people in that study. These numbers are based on averages and percentages of large groups of people; your response may be similar or different depending on where in the spectrum (or *off* the spectrum) of responses that occurred in the study your own response falls.

Charts and Graphs

Charts and graphs are a way of depicting numbers as pictures to make them easier to understand. Most people find this type of visualization helpful. The most common types you'll find are:

PIE CHART

This diagram is an easy way of representing proportions. The "pie" is represented by a circle, and each "slice" in the pie represents a portion of the whole. For example, if we were to draw a pie chart to represent the different number of hours people took to fall asleep in the double-caffeine condition, it would look like this:

Time to Sleep for Double-Caffeine Subjects

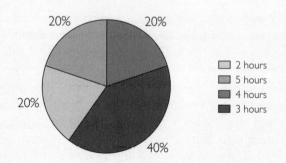

BAR CHART

Also sometimes called a bar graph, this is a single chart with a series of horizontal or vertical bars that represent different values. This diagram can make it easy to see differences among various experimental conditions because you can compare the height or length of the various bars to one another. For example, we can chart the number of people who fell asleep (represented on the y-axis or the vertical direction) after a particular amount of time (represented on the x-axis or horizontal direction) by the amount of caffeine they got. Our three different caffeine conditions are represented by three different color-coded bars. With this type of chart, it is easy to see how the different caffeine conditions affected sleep time. For example, if you look at the third set of bars, this shows that one person in the decaf condition fell asleep after two hours, three people in the regular coffee condition, and two people in the double-strength condition. (The first bar goes up as high as "1" as measured on the left axis, the second bar goes as high as "3," and the third bar goes as high as "2." That all three of these bars are clustered together means that they are measurements taken at the same point—here, at two hours to fall asleep.)

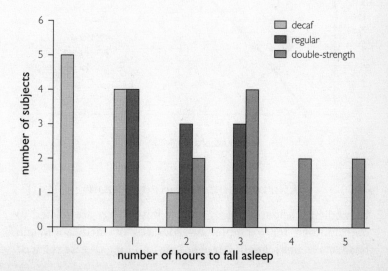

LINE GRAPHS

These types of diagrams use lines to allow you to see trends or progress clearly. Each condition is represented by a line that has various data points through time. In our example, each of our caffeine conditions would get its own line, and the number of subjects who had fallen asleep by a given hour would be tracked throughout the night. If you follow any one of the lines, you can see the effect of that condition. For example, in the decaf condition, most subjects fell asleep immediately, a few took a little longer, but everyone was asleep after two hours. But in the double-strength condition, no one fell asleep quickly, and some people didn't fall asleep until 4 or 5 A.M. The regular caffeine group is in the middle, with no one falling asleep quickly, but everyone asleep by 3 A.M.

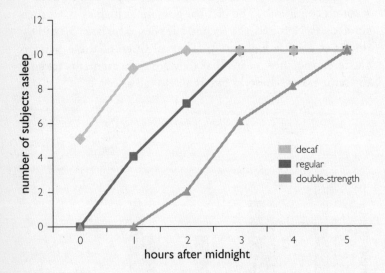

Correlation and Regression

In medicine, scientists like to know how things are related to one another, for example: Are dosages of medication and headache relief related? Are smoking and lung disease related?

Are caffeine and sleeplessness related? One of the ways to tell that is through *correlation*. We can just look at the numbers in our coffee experiment and see that there seems to be a relationship between caffeine and sleeplessness, that the more caffeine a subject drank, the longer they were likely to stay awake. In a large study, the trends would be much more difficult to see, so scientists need to rely on statistical analysis to determine correlation.

Correlations come in two types, positive and negative. When two quantities are positively correlated, large values of one quantity are associated with large values of the other quantity. Thus in our experiment the amount of caffeine consumed and the length of time before the subject fell asleep are positively correlated. When large values of one quantity are associated with small values of the other, we say that the quantities are negatively correlated. In that case, we might expect to find that the amount of caffeine consumed and the hours of sleep that night are negatively correlated; the larger amounts of caffeine correspond with fewer hours of sleep for that subject.

A statistic called the correlation coefficient, usually represented by the variable r, summarizes the correlation of two variables. This coefficient takes on values between -1 and 1, representing the strength and direction of the correlation. If r is negative, then the correlation is negative. If r is positive, then the correlation is positive. When r has a large magnitude (it is near 1 or -1), the correlation is called strong because the data are very nearly linearly related. This means that if the data were plotted (as in a line graph), a single straight line would pass near or through all of the points. When r has a small magnitude (it is near 0), the correlation is called weak. This means that the large values of one quantity can be found with either large or small values of the other quantity. In the coffee experiment we would have a weak correlation if some of the subjects who drank double-strength coffee fell asleep right away while some of the decaf-drinkers tossed and turned for several hours. Sometimes the direction of the correlation is clear and researchers discuss r^2, which gives just the strength of the correlation. (An r^2 near zero means the correlation is weak, near 1 is strong.)

Scientists can perform a certain statistical analysis called a *regression* to determine which straight line (or sometimes a more complicated mathematical graph) best fits the data, and how good the fit is to the data. If the correlation is strong, the regression line can be used to make predictions. For instance, if researchers found a regression for the hours you would be sleepless based on your caffeine consumption, you could use it to manage your sleeplessness by controlling how much caffeine you drank. (Of course, most of us find that other factors besides the amount of caffeine we drink contributes to how much trouble we have going to sleep.)

It is important to note that just because two things are corre-lated doesn't mean that one necessarily *causes* the other. There is always the possibility that there are other undiscovered con-nections between the factors. For example, during a cholera epidemic in Russia, the government sent doctors to the worst-affected areas. The peasants in one province discussed the situ-ation in their villages and noticed that there was a strong positive correlation between the number of doctors in a village and the incidence of cholera. Reversing the direction of causa-tion, they assumed that the doctors were causing the cholera outbreaks, and proceeded to murder the doctors. This story makes clear the dangers of misjudging correlation for causa-tion!

Significance, Probability, and Confidence

There is always a certain amount of unavoidable error in the data gathered in an experiment. And as we discussed at the beginning of this chapter, it is very important for medical stud-ies to account for the inevitable individual variations in responses. After all, not everyone who smokes gets cancer, and not everyone who drank the double-caffeine coffee stayed up five hours. Since people are different, they react differently to any given set of variables, treatments, or experimental conditions. The uncertainty this causes is taken into consideration in any statistical analysis.

Any statistical result reported in a medical journal must meet minimal standards for *significance* (evidence so strong that it is not likely to be due to chance), so you know that the conclusions being drawn are likely to be correct. In general, medical science follows the tradition that an experimental result is considered *significant* if the *probability* that the result would happen by chance is less than 5 in 100. And the experimental results would be considered *very significant* or *highly significant* if the probability that the result would occur by chance was less than 1 in 100. If you read the results section of a medical journal article, you'll read about various kinds of statistical tests that were performed on the data, and then in parentheses, you'll see a *p-value* where the *p* stands for the probability that determines significance. For example, if you see: (p ≤ .05), you know that the relationship tested was significant, with a probability less than or equal to 5 out of 100 that it occurred by chance. The smaller the number in a p-value (it isn't unusual to see p ≤ .01, p ≤ .001, or p ≤ .0001) the stronger the effect, as tested in the experiment. Sometimes a paper will report a p-value of "marginal significance" or "approaching significance," such as if the probability were slightly greater than 5 in 100 (e.g.: p ≤ .08). This is often reported as a signal to other researchers that there *might* be something important to investigate, but that significance level wasn't reached in this particular experiment. This often happens if the subject pool for the study was not quite large enough to smooth out the individual variability that might hide the effect.

Another related term you'll often see in medical articles is *confidence interval* and *level of confidence*. For any given set of numbers generated in an experiment, there is a certain amount of error possible that cannot be controlled due to individual variability or measurement error. For example, in our coffee study, there is always the possibility that some people incorrectly reported the time they fell asleep. This would give us a different mean than if we had access to the true times. When reporting medical results, scientists may give the confidence interval, or confidence limits, which define a range of numbers within which the scientists are reasonably certain (based on statistics) the true mean exists. They will report their level of confidence (usually 95 percent or higher) that the true mean lies somewhere in that confidence interval. The width of this interval depends on two factors. The first is variation: The more individual variation and measurement error is associated with this quantity, the wider its confidence interval will be. The second is the size of the subject pool for the study: The more subjects tested, the narrower the confidence interval will be. A well-defined and adequately funded study will begin with a large enough subject pool to compensate for even a widely variable quantity, and give a confidence interval that is useful. But even the best researchers conduct studies where their plans fall apart. For instance, many subjects unexpectedly leave the study, or the variability of a critical quantity turns out to be much larger than anyone expected. Good researchers will explain what went wrong and why, and follow-up studies will correct these mistakes. Usually, you can accept a mean and not worry about its confidence interval, but sometimes, particularly in cutting-edge or controversial research or work that has trouble getting funding, it pays to study these error estimates carefully.

Risk, Relative Risk, Risk Factors

As a patient, you'll hear a lot about various kinds of risks. The word itself sounds frightening, but remember, some risk numbers may be in your favor—it's just another way of talking about variability in different people's experiences.

• *Risk* is typically defined as the probability that a particular event or outcome will occur. (For example, in our experiment, drinking caffeine could be said to lead to an increased *risk* of sleeplessness. Also, some studies have shown that getting regular exercise decreases your *risk* of certain types of cancers.)

• *Risk factors* are conditions or situations that are associated with increased chances of developing a condition, illness, or disease. (For example, smoking is a risk factor for lung cancer.)

• *Lifetime risk* refers to the probability of a particular event or outcome occurring over the entire course of a typical lifetime. (For example, it has been said that women have a 50 percent chance or a one-in-two lifetime risk of dying of heart disease.) This is a very tricky type of risk to calculate, and it does not easily apply to individuals.

• *Absolute risk* is a specific term that basically means the total risk of a particular outcome occurring as the result of some other intervention. It is, for example, the total risk of a particular side effect faced by people who take a certain drug. (For example, it may be that individuals who are exposed to certain chemicals face an *absolute risk* of 2 cancers per 500,000 people exposed.) It does not take into account the risk of the same outcome faced by people who did not take the drug, undergo the procedure, or face the event.

• *Relative risk* is a term you are likely to see often, and it is the term that is likely to be most confusing. To understand this topic, consider this example: We all have some risk of developing heart disease. This is called the "background" risk because it is lurking there for everyone. Since diabetes is a specific risk factor for heart disease, people who are diagnosed with diabetes have an increased risk of heart disease *over the background risk*. Relative risk would describe the additional risk of heart disease faced by people with diabetes beyond the background risk we all face.

Specifically, then, relative risk is the ratio between the number of health outcomes expected of people who are exposed to some outside factor, and the number of health outcomes expected in a group of people who were not exposed. (The outside factors can be anything that increases a risk, including other illness, surgery, medication, or diet.) It is expressed as a decimal. A relative risk of 1.0 means no additional risk beyond what would be typical "background" risk. A relative risk of 2.0

means that the risk is twice as large as background risk. On the other hand, a relative risk of 0.50 means that the medication or event cut the risk in half from what would be typical.

It's always important to look at relative risk numbers in context. A large relative risk may actually mean very little actual risk. For example, if the *relative risk* of having an ischemic stroke is 5.0 among people who take a particular medication, that means that those patients have a risk of stroke that is five times greater than the risk faced by a person not taking the medication. That sounds like a huge number. But if the actual risk is only one in a million, it means that people who take the medication have five times that risk, or a five-in-a-million risk of ischemic stroke. That's still a very rare event. On the other hand, if the actual risk is 1 in 10, then taking the medication would increase the risk to 5 in 10 or 50 percent. That would be something to be concerned about.

16. Shared Decision Making

We make decisions about our health every day. Every time you choose to take a walk, cook a nutritious meal, take your medication as directed, test your blood glucose levels, or keep a doctor's appointment, you've made a decision that affects your health and well-being.

Generally, these decisions are easy to make, and their overall impact feels minor because they are so commonplace. But in fact, these small decisions can be quite significant. Consider this: A major cause of blindness is the eye disease glaucoma, which can be controlled with prescription eye medication, but studies show that less than half of all patients who received prescription eye drops that could save their sight used the medication regularly. The single decision to skip a dose of medication may not have much of an effect, but with enough "skipping," the overall health effects can be serious.

Medical decisions become more difficult to make when the effects are more immediate and more profound. For example, diseases or treatments that are potentially life-threatening require a more in-depth decision-making process.

In the not-so-distant paternalistic past, doctors would make decisions for their patients, often without offering them alternatives. If you are over age forty, you may have heard stories of women who went into the hospital for a breast biopsy and woke up with a breast removed. The thinking was that if cancer was detected, the course of treatment that offered the best chance of survival was mastectomy, so the doctor did the job. The women were not usually asked whether they wanted their breasts removed, nor were they given time to get used to the idea.

Now, improvements in medical knowledge and technology make patient participation in the decision-making process a near-necessity. This might seem counterintuitive: If we know more about diseases and treatments, shouldn't we become *more* certain about what the "right" choice would be for any given disease? Unfortunately, no. Imagine that you are just beginning to learn how to cook, and your first lesson is how to make spaghetti. If all you know how to cook is spaghetti, then you pretty much know what you'll have for dinner tonight, tomorrow night, and the night after that. You have no other choice. But as you learn to cook more dishes, your choices expand and the decision of what to have for dinner becomes more difficult. Similarly, the more options there are for treating a disease, the more room there is for choice.

In medical circles, the problem is made more complex by the fact that every treatment option has risks as well as benefits. There are consequences for every option. A drug that you took successfully a few years ago may cause an allergic reaction if you take it again this year; the same operation that saves a man's life may also leave him with constant pain; the chemotherapy that puts one patient into remission may permanently damage the immune system of another. And who has to live with these consequences? The patient. So more and more physicians and medical ethicists now believe that the patient should have more say in which treatment is chosen. Yes, doctors always try to do what's best for their patients, but in the end it is the patient who is most affected—for better or for worse—by the choice of treatment. It is in your best interest that you participate in making the decision about what treatments you receive.

Decision-Making Basics

First, don't worry, *you're not in this alone.* Just because you participate in decision making doesn't mean that the doctor will simply list your options and force you to make a life-or-death decision. (If your doctor does, find a new doctor!)

"The key word is 'partnership,'" says Judith A. Erlen, Ph.D., R.N., professor and associate director of the Center for Research and Chronic Disorders at the University of Pittsburgh School of Nursing. "That's really what you want to have happen. You want to be a partner in the decision making."

When it comes to making a medical decision, the doctor and the patient each have areas of expertise. Doctors have experience and technical information: the biology of disease, how treatments work, what the risks and benefits are, what scientific studies have shown about the success rates, and how other patients have fared. Patients have personal information: the values they hold, their beliefs about their illnesses, their plans for the future, and their likes and dislikes. By sharing what they know, discussing the risks and benefits of all alternatives, and focusing on the patient's needs and expectations, physicians and patients can work together to come to the best decision for each patient.

Let me repeat that last phrase because it is critically important: *Physicians and patients can work together to come to the best decision for each patient.* The decision that was right for your uncle or your next-door neighbor may be very different from the decision that is right for you. Decisions that affect your health and your life depend strongly on the personal factors you feel are important. For example, some people who are diagnosed with cancer have an immediate reaction of "get that cancer out of me." They want surgery—and fast. But what if the cancer is so extremely slow-growing that it may not cause problems for another fifteen years? And what if there is a 50 percent chance that surgery to remove it will cause urinary incontinence? Different people have different judgments about what factors are important. Some patients will still want immediate surgery, even with the risk of incontinence, because they cannot stand the thought of cancer in their bodies. Others will find the prospect of possible incontinence intolerable and will live with the cancer, hoping that it remains slow-growing. Both of these choices are "right" if they are in line with the values and beliefs of the patients making the decision.

Second, rest assured that *no doctor will let you make a decision that will have significant repercussions without letting you know exactly what you're getting into.* For example: Medically speaking, the most effective treatment for many types of cancer is chemotherapy. It isn't pleasant, and there are quite a few possible side effects (including hair loss), but chemotherapy can, in many cases, extend life or put cancer into remission. Yet there are patients who feel that the loss of their hair is too great a sacrifice and choose not to take chemotherapy drugs. Physicians will not simply say, "OK, whatever you want." They will try to educate these patients, listen to their objections, and make sure that they understand that they may be risking death for the sake of their hair.

"Doctors really try to help patients understand, but there's a fine line," says Dr. Erlen. "You don't want to coerce a patient into a making a decision, either. You need to guide people . . . without putting words in somebody's mouth." Some physicians will tell patients that they should find a new doctor if they refuse the treatment that is most medically justified. The final choice is still the patient's, but a good doctor won't let a potentially harmful choice go unchallenged.

Third, it's important to understand that the science of medicine and the science of medical decision making are continually evolving and improving. Doctors don't know everything about diseases and treatments because not everything has been discovered yet. Just think, the penicillin we take for granted today wasn't widely available until the 1940s. Until then, people died of complications from simple infections. Doctors can offer only what is available, either in terms of information or options. This means that *you may be asked to make a decision without having all the information you would like to have.* There is a very good possibility that no one will be able to tell you which treatment will definitely cure you, if a cure is even possible, or how long the cure will last.

"You cannot promise somebody that [a treatment] is going to work all the time," says Dr. Erlen. "There is a lot of uncertainty. Even though you have knowledge, in many instances that knowledge is not going to be 100 percent. There's going to be pieces missing. That's a given."

This will make the decision more difficult, but it is still possible to come to the best decision for you. We make decisions based on limited or incomplete information all the time. "Think back over decisions you've made in the past," says Dr. Erlen. "You probably weren't 100 percent certain about some of those decisions. Were you 100 percent certain about the person you were marrying? Or about the last car you bought? You could have bought a lemon. . . . There's a certain amount of uncertainty in many, many decisions that we make. Once you realize that, you can begin to transfer that process over to making medical decisions."

Finally, *you won't have to decide everything.* Although many physicians recommend including patient preferences in all phases of medical care, there are some things you won't have a choice about. For example, you won't have to decide what your diagnosis is, or what the possible treatment options are, or how the treatments progress.

Sometimes the treatments are clear—if you have a ruptured appendix, the appendix must be surgically removed if you want to survive. No choice. Other decisions that may be out of your hands have to do with the specifics of treatment that occur after you make a more general decision. For example, you may decide that you want surgery, but you won't be able to decide where the doctor will make the incision.

Different Levels and Types of Medical Decisions

Not all medical decisions are made the same way, or with the same information, or for the same reasons. When patients are faced with the need to make medical decisions, it is important for them to understand that there are different critical aspects that play an important role in the process. Decision-making expert Dennis J. Mazur, M.D., Ph.D., professor of medicine at Oregon Health Sciences University and chairman of the Institutional Review Board of the Department of Veterans Affairs Medical Center in Portland, Oregon, has outlined eight of these aspects, or dimensions, of shared decision making.

"The one exciting opportunity patients and physicians have in each of the dimensions . . . is learning, understanding, and optimizing each other's experiences in the area for the ultimate goal of optimized shared decision making," says Dr. Mazur.

Each dimension comes into play for every decision, but in varying degrees. By understanding where you and your situation fall in each of these dimensions, you will be able to adjust your approach to making medical decisions:

1. URGENCIES AND TIME CONSTRAINTS

In extreme emergency situations, there may not be time for a patient to become involved in making a medical decision. Similarly, if a patient is unconscious, in extreme pain, or otherwise affected by illness, he or she may not be lucid enough to participate in the process. In these cases, the decisions will be made by the physician after discussions with the patient's family and with due consideration of any advance directives the patient may have completed beforehand. In addition, the hospital's chaplain, medical ethicist, or clinical ethics committee may be called in for perspectives should there be enough time to allow such deliberations without compromising patient care in the emergent or urgent situation. At the other extreme, decision making can be more leisurely. For example, the patient just diagnosed with mild hypertension (without signs of any end-organ hypertensive damage to his or her eyes, heart, kidneys, or brain) has time to search for information, have multiple discussions with doctors and other health professionals, try diet and lifestyle changes, and consider the side-effect profiles of different medications before actually starting a drug regimen. *Ask your doctor how urgent your situation is so you know how much time you can safely take to make your decision.*

2. DECISION WEIGHTS

Some decisions are heavier, or more serious, than others. Some are life-and-death decisions, where simple survival is at stake. Others are serious quality-of-life decisions (e.g., involving pain control) in which the options revolve around how to make the patient as comfortable as possible within the constraints of the illness. Still others are relatively "light" decisions involving less critical aspects of care, such as whether to have a hip replacement immediately or wait a few years and continue on pain medication for the hip discomfort. *All medical decisions carry consequences, but more serious potential consequences demand a higher level of awareness and consideration. Risks and benefits for serious outcomes (survival and quality of life) are important information for making a rational decision.*

3. LEVELS OF RISK AND CHANCES OF BENEFIT

Some medical interventions are riskier than others, and some patients have higher risk because of their fragile physical and psychological states. *For each option, the level of risk and the chance of benefit in the patient's particular case should be clearly defined by the physician.* In generating these estimates in your particular case, Dr. Mazur notes that the physician needs to rely on his or her own training and clinical experience, the opinion of expert physicians, and a firm understanding of the current medical scientific literature.

4. LEVELS OF PHYSICIAN EXPERIENCE

How many cases like yours has your doctor treated? As discussed in chapter 11, the more cases a doctor or hospital treats, the better your chance of a positive outcome because your doctor has more experience with the disease, its presentation, and its behavior over time in different people under different treatments or management strategies. For common disorders, such as high cholesterol or hypertension, virtually any doctor has likely treated thousands of cases, and the treatment options may be relatively standard (although they still may be debated in terms of what is in fact the "best" approach to treatment in a particular patient). On the other hand, some diseases are so rare that no one can be considered an expert. *To optimize your treatment, seek a physician or hospital that treats a great number of patients with your type of illness. For rare disorders, if no expert is available, seek a physician who is willing to go the extra mile to do additional information searches and gather the knowledge necessary to offer you sound medical advice.*

5. LEVELS OF "NUMERACY" AMONG PATIENTS

We all differ in our abilities to understand and work with numbers. Physicians communicate with other physicians using numbers, fractions, percentages, odds ratios, and other numerical expressions as they discuss and deliberate about the statistics involved in a particular medical decision. Patients, on the other hand, often prefer to communicate using words such as "probable," "rare," or "possible." Very different meanings can be assigned to these words, however, which can lead to miscommunication between physician and patient. For example, if a "rare" chance of dying to you means one out of a million, but to your doctor it means one out of 100, you are talking about very different risks. (See chapter 17 for some common definitions of numbers and statistics.) *If you understand numbers relatively well, ask your doctor to use them whenever possible. Whenever you hear verbal probability terms (such as "rare" or "likely"), ask your doctor what he or she means by them, as specifically as possible.*

6. LEVELS OF COMMUNICATION SKILLS AMONG PHYSICIANS

Different doctors have different abilities to communicate risks, benefits, treatments, and other aspects of your illness. Specialists (such as cardiologists, oncologists, nephrologists, endocrinologists) can explain the nuances and specifics of your particular illness related to their area of specialty well because their focus is on a smaller set of medical conditions and disease processes related to their specialty. General physicians, on the other hand, often have a broader base of medical knowledge and can often help patients better understand and place into context overall risk, taking into account all aspects of the patient's health. This is especially true in relation to the patient with multiple medical conditions on multiple medications. In an ideal world, we could bring all the specialists and generalists together in one room for three hours and ask all the questions we want. Unfortunately, we don't have that luxury of time. *Address specialty questions to the specialist, and general questions to your primary care physician.* Oftentimes, the specialist will ask you to talk over the perspectives he or she offers with your primary care physician. In addition, your primary care physician can often help you understand more clearly what the specialist is saying in light of your overall health and medical conditions. Whenever possible, take some time to do an information search on your own to save time in the specialist and primary care physicians' offices for the truly critical questions.

7. LEVELS OF SCIENTIFIC EVIDENCE

For some medical decisions, high-quality research (specifically, multicenter randomized controlled clinical trials) has been done, and the results relate directly to your condition and treatment. (See chapter 9 for more information on the different types of research studies; and see "Clinical Trials," page 278.) With strong scientific results, the physician can interpret the results for the patient and offer a specific treatment with more confidence. Without high-quality studies, doctors can offer only their perspectives based on their own clinical experiences and the clinical experiences of a group of experts. Anecdotal evidence (evidence based on the reported experiences of a handful of patients) is not considered good scientific evidence. But, in some cases, it may be all the evidence that is available at that particular time because high-quality research studies have not been started, or such studies are still in the process of being completed and interpreted. *Ask your doctor*

*what types of research studies have been done and how he or she
interprets the studies in general and in relation to you, the patient.
If no high-quality studies have been done, ask your physician what
expert clinical opinions are available, and which of those opinions
he or she supports.* Obviously, the decision-making process is
easier if the treatment has been studied in high-quality clinical
trials.

8. CONSTRAINTS

Various constraints can exist that limit or bar shared decision
making. For example, if you live in Oregon, but the only expert
who deals with your illness is based in New York, you may have
difficulty gaining access to the expert. (In the future, consultations via the Internet and telemedicine will become more common, but these approaches also need to be systematically
studied in multicenter randomized controlled trials to determine their risks and benefits to the patient.) Also, there may be
cost constraints. For example, health insurance constraints may
prevent a physician from offering a patient the full range of
drugs for the patient's medical condition. *Talk with your physician about any constraints in your treatment decisions. There may
be ways of overcoming or compensating for the difficulties if everyone is aware of them.*

Putting It All Together

Ideally, we should be making medical decisions throughout our
lives, starting from the time we can decide which color ban-
dage we want on a cut. Early practice with simpler and more
innocuous decisions can prepare us for the big decisions we'll
have to make one day. Since people make decisions in their
own way, based on their illness, the treatment options presented, their values and dreams, there is no easy step-by-step
process for making medical decisions. There are, however, some
general guidelines and points to consider that may be helpful:

Take your time: Ask your doctor how much time you have
to decide about treatment. Very few medical problems require

urgent action or decision making. Usually there is some time available for you to review all your options, do an information search, talk with professionals and other patients, and finally come to a decision.

"Usually what happens is that when somebody's diagnosed, they're in a state of shock," says Susan Love, M.D., director of the nonprofit Susan Love Breast Cancer Foundation and coauthor of *Dr. Susan Love's Breast Book* and *Dr. Susan Love's Hormone Book*. "For the first twenty-four hours, they really can't hear anything or do anything. But that then goes away . . . just hold on until that shock goes away."

Ask about risks, benefits, and outcomes in numbers: Before any decision can be made, it's important to understand exactly what the decision entails. Hearing about outcomes in terms of numbers can make a decision easier because they eliminate the ambiguity inherent in using terms like "rare," "probable," and "possible." Numbers based on solid research data can help you define exactly what the possibilities are. It is a very different thing to decide between "treatment with surgery and treatment with medication" than it is to decide between "surgery with a 90 percent chance of success (and 10 percent chance of failure) and medication with a 25 percent chance of success (and a 75 percent chance of failure)."

Pay attention to how numbers are being presented: Dr. Mazur notes that "Even when numbers are used in a patient-physician dialogue, the way that the numerical information is presented to patients may also unfairly influence their choice of treatments. This is particularly true when numbers are presented in too-abbreviated a fashion. For example, when, in a fast-paced discussion of risks and benefits, surgical data is provided in terms of 'survival only,' the patient may fail to recognize that there is also 'risk of dying or mortality risk' associated with that survival statistic. That is, a 90 percent chance of survival in the short term (during a medical or surgical intervention or within thirty days after that intervention) has with it a 10 percent chance of dying in the short term."

Your physician will help you place the numbers in a con-

text: Your doctor should be able to help put words like "rare" or "probable" into numbers. But Dr. Mazur also notes that physicians can then help you understand the numbers and place them in context. Physicians can read a research study and place an individual patient within the overall context of the study by asking questions like "How similar (or different) is my patient to the patients studied in the clinical trial?" And based on that assessment, they assign risk and benefit numbers. For treatments or diseases that have not been well studied, the physician can look at the experiences of other doctors as written up in medical journals and make assessments from that information. The assessments in that case won't be as well-founded as those based on clinical trials, but they can still provide a basis for beginning to talk seriously about risks and benefits.

Note: Some people stop listening when numbers are discussed because they are not used to hearing them or using them in general conversation. If you find these types of conversations confusing or stressful, ask your doctor to write down the numbers and what they mean so you can review them again in the relative calm and privacy of your home. If you still find them confusing, ask the doctor if there is another health professional, such as a nurse or physician's assistant, who might be able to take the time to talk you through it.

Consider your values: By values, experts mean those personal thoughts, feelings, and beliefs that you hold about your body and your life. For example, Dupuytren's contracture is a painless condition in which there is a thickening of the tissue under the skin of the palm. This causes, for example, the fourth and/or fifth fingers to contract, bending toward the palm, in a way that cannot be straightened again. If you had this problem, would you be willing to endure delicate hand surgery to correct the condition? It depends on your values. The answer would likely be yes if the disorder prevented you from playing a musical instrument you enjoyed, or if you were relatively young, or if your livelihood depended on full use of your hands. The answer might be no, however, if only the pinkie finger was involved and caused no great difference in your daily activities, or if you were in your nineties, or if you were terribly afraid of surgery.

"Information is important, but values are also really important," says Dr. Erlen. "People can start by asking themselves, 'What's important in my life? Where would I like to be in five years? What kinds of goals do I have? What do I want to do when I retire?' The context, of course, will change depending on life circumstances, such as age, and whether the patient does or does not have a family. The only way you come face-to-face with your values is to spend some time asking yourself some hard questions."

Sometimes you can help clarify your values by listening to other people tell their stories by participating in a self-help group, talking with other patients or reading books by survivors. You can learn what their thought processes were, how they came to make the decisions they made, and what the effect has been on their lives. You can begin to think, "Do I see things in the same way? Why don't I see them in the same way?"

After you have a good idea of what you value, try to determine how those values agree or contrast with your doctors' values. Make sure your doctors understand your point of view, and if they offer conflicting points of view, ask why they feel that way. They may present some information you hadn't thought of before, or they may simply have a different set of values.

Understand that fear is common and can be dealt with: Some people make even the most monumental decisions quickly and easily. Others can become paralyzed by the prospect of deciding their own medical treatment. "Regret . . . may be a reason some patients want to give up their decision-making authority to their physicians," says Dr. Mazur. "The patient does not want to experience the regret of making the wrong decision on his or her own. But physicians also can experience regret when they take on all the decision-making responsibility. . . . In addition, patients can later regret giving the decision to the physician, especially if the outcome is not what the patient expected or hoped for."

Your best chance for limiting fear and regret is to understand the potential outcomes and their likelihood, and then talk with your physician about your fears. The fears themselves may help you and your doctor decide the type of treatment that might be better for you. For example, if your greatest fear is that you'll be partially paralyzed after surgery, you and your doctor may decide to try a nonsurgical treatment first.

Ask questions: Think of what you would like to have happen, then talk with your doctor about the best ways to accomplish it. This lets your doctor know some of your values, concerns, and preferences, and offers a starting position to begin a conversation. Some people find it easier to understand and use information to make decisions if they ask *what if.* "What if I decide to have the surgery . . . what is likely to happen?" "What if I wait until after my daughter's wedding before starting treatment . . . would that be harmful?" You should feel free to ask any question that might help you make the decision, but you should also understand that the doctor may not have answers. Even if you don't get all the answers you want, at least you will have defined exactly what is known and not known about your situation.

Get a second, or third, opinion for other perspectives: Just as every patient has a different set of values, different doctors will have different treatment preferences. "We know that with many treatments and procedures in the country, what the doctor recommends . . . and what you hear is the optimal treatment . . . may very well depend on where you live," says Michael J. Barry, M.D., chief of general medicine at Massachusetts General Hospital in Boston. "If the patient is getting a treatment recommendation that seems to be clashing with their preferences, where the recommendations say to pick surgical therapy but [the patient has] significant concerns about a potential side effect, then that's the ideal time for a second opinion. If what the first doctor is telling them really seems to fit with what they've learned about the condition and their own preferences, then I think a second opinion may be less important."

It can also be helpful to get a second opinion from someone in a different discipline. As a general rule, surgeons recommend surgery and radiation therapists recommend radiation. If you are deciding between surgery and radiation as treatments, talk to both types of specialists to make sure you get both opinions presented fairly.

Make a list of pros and cons for each option: It may sound like a cliché, but seeing the positive and negative aspects of each treatment written out in black and white can sometimes help make the decision clearer. Include everything, medical probabilities as well as how the treatment will affect the things you value.

Ask your doctor if decision aids are available: As physicians and researchers realized the importance of involving patients in medical decisions, they began to consider ways to help the process. It is difficult for physicians to find the time to sit down with every patient for a considerable length of time to discuss all facets of disease information, treatment options, and values judgments. Patients who can gather their own information are better prepared to make a decision, but they also often have multiple questions that need to be answered before coming to a final decision. And not all patients are skillful information gatherers.

To fill this need, different groups are developing various types of decision aids. These health communication tools take many forms, including interactive videodiscs, videotapes, decision boards, and flip-charts with audiotapes. They are designed to explain current disease and treatment information clearly, summarize risks and benefits, report scientific evidence, provide a variety of clinical perspectives, and help patients see the "big picture" in a way that is not overwhelming. In some cases, patients have the opportunity to hear other patients tell why they chose the treatment they did and what their lives have been like since then.

The use of decision aids is only in its infancy, but it promises to be an important part of medical care in the future. "My prediction is that [this will expand] in the next five years or so," says Annette O'Connor, Ph.D., R.N., professor at the University of Ottawa School of Nursing and Faculty of Medicine and senior investigator at the Ottawa Hospital Loeb Health Research Institute in Ontario, Canada. Health maintenance organizations are beginning to look at patient satisfaction with counseling and decision support as one of their "report card" issues. In order to score well, organizations will have to find ways to improve counseling, and decision aids seem like the perfect tool: They are simple to use, easy for the consumer to understand, and initial research has shown that they seem to work. Some researchers have found that approximately half of the patients who are undecided about treatment are helped in their decision by the decision aids. For patients who already have a preference, the decision aids tend to confirm their choices, making them more confident. "Everyone gets more informed," says Dr. O'Connor. "And a lot of people feel much more comfortable with their decision, having used these tools."

Currently, decision aids have been created for only a small subset of diseases, generally those where there is a considerable "gray zone" for decision making—when it really depends on the person's health situation and personal values. These include prostate cancer, benign prostatic hyperplasia, benign uterine conditions, breast cancer, lower back pain, mild hypertension, hormone replacement therapy, and ischemic heart disease. No doubt more diseases and conditions will be covered in the future.

Decision aids are not meant to be a "homework assignment" that you take home, complete, and come back with a fully formed decision. These tools are best used in conjunction with a good doctor-patient partnership. "I consider decision aids as tools for preparing you for a fruitful discussion," says Dr. O'Connor. "Nobody wants to make a decision on a video screen." What the decision aid does is allow you to think through the decision and start formulating your own ideas without actually committing yourself to the choice. Then you can go back and discuss your possible decision with your doctor.

Since the decision aids need to be updated frequently to incorporate the latest information, they are expensive to produce. Only a few doctors have access to them, but your doctor or health insurance company may be able to point you to a source that will have them. (*Note:* Always ask when the decision aid was last updated or reviewed. The best companies review information every few months and make changes when new information becomes available.) Some medical centers may have access, and some insurance companies cover the cost of decision aids.

One of the most recognized and respected organizations that produces decision aids is the Foundation for Informed Medical Decision Making (in partnership with Health Dialog). You can find out more about which decision aids they produce, order a decision aid, and find out whether your insurance will cover it by contacting Health Dialog directly (by phone at 617-854-7440) or checking their website: http://www.healthdialog.com.

Other excellent sources of decision aids are the Loeb Health Research Institute and the Cochrane Library. Dr. O'Connor and her colleagues at the Loeb Health Research Institute in Ottawa have created some decision aids and are making them available free of charge online at http://www.lri.ca/programs/ceu/ohdec/decision_aids.htm. This website also provides related publications and links to other related sites. The Cochrane Library is an electronic publication designed to supply high-quality medical evidence and reviews. It is published quarterly on CD-ROM and the Internet, and is distributed on a subscription basis. For more information about what they have available, see the website at http://www.update-software.com/cochrane/cochrane-frame.html. (If this Web address changes, search under keywords "Cochrane Library" on your search engine.) Abstracts of the reviews are available without charge on the same website.

Talk with other people: Get the perspectives of friends, family members, other patients, and other health professionals. Consider their positions, listen to their experiences, and use them to test how you feel about the decision. Remember that the final decision is yours, and should be based on how you feel about it in the context of risks, benefits, and values.

Trust yourself: You are the only person who knows how you feel and think about your life, your illness, and your treatment. With the help of a good physician who will act as your health care partner, you are capable of making the medical decision that is best for you.

CLINICAL TRIALS

One of the decisions you may have to (or want to) make during your treatment is whether you should participate in a clinical trial. As with all medical decisions, you'll need to evaluate the type of trial, what it is studying, the financial and time costs, risks and benefits, and your own values before coming to a conclusion.

What Are Clinical Trials?

A clinical trial is basically a fancy name for scientific research in which a physician or clinical investigator uses human subjects to study new drugs, disease treatments, or disease prevention methods. Because clinical trials are often used to prove the value of a new treatment and justify adding it to the medical arsenal, the studies must be reviewed by the Institutional Review Board (IRB) of the institution sponsoring the trial to make sure they are well-designed. This review process also ensures that the people who participate won't end up being mere "guinea pigs" in the experiment, and that precautions are taken to limit the risks.

The research that goes into a clinical trial usually starts long before patients become involved. Typically, many years of work have already been done to assess how well the new medication might work and how safe it will likely be by conducting experiments in test tubes or on laboratory animals. If enough evidence points to a potential benefit in humans, a clinical trial is designed.

There are three stages, or "phases," to a clinical trial. Not all trials complete all three phases. If the new treatment being tested is shown to be unsafe or ineffective, the trial will stop.

- *Phase 1 clinical trials* investigate how a drug (or treatment) should be given and whether it is safe for humans. For example, a phase 1 clinical trial might look at how much of a drug should be given, how often, and in what form (by mouth, by nasal spray, by injection). Very few patients are enrolled—sometimes fewer than twenty. Limited information is gathered about whether the treatment works. If the treatment appears safe, phase 2 trials can be conducted.

- *Phase 2 clinical trials* begin to investigate whether the treatment works in humans, and continues to look at the safety of the treatment. A small number of patients are enrolled. If the treatment seems to be effective, phase 3 trials can be conducted. If no effect is seen, the trial is stopped.

- *Phase 3 clinical trials* compare the new treatment to the best standard care in current use. These studies usually enroll large numbers of patients—often thousands from multiple medical centers across the country. In order to ensure that similar types of patients receive the various treatments under investigation, the participants are usually randomly selected to receive either the new treatment or the current standard treatment. Because so many participants are needed for a phase 3 trial, this is the type for which you are most likely to be recruited.

There are advantages and disadvantages to participating in a clinical trial. The advantages are that your care is carefully monitored by a medical team that has an investment in your well-being, you have a chance to receive state-of-the-art treatment, you will receive *at least* the best standard care, you have the potential for improved outcome, and you have the opportunity to contribute to the body of medical knowledge that may one day save the lives of future patients.

The disadvantages are that the potential toxicities of the treatment are unknown (in phase 1 trials), you and your doctor won't be able to decide the treatment you receive (your treatment will be based on random assignment [phase 3 trials only]), the trial may require additional expense and time investment, and some patients don't like the thought of being part of an experiment.

Deciding on a Clinical Trial

As with all medical decisions, you should make your decision to participate in a clinical trial only after thoroughly investigating the scope of the treatment, understanding all your treatment options, and consulting your physician. Questions you should ask before volunteering that can guide your decision are:

- What will I get out of it? How might it help my condition? Will my participation simply help other people without direct benefit to me?
- What if I don't participate, what other treatment options are there?
- Why is this being offered to me? Is there something unique about my condition that means this is a better option for me than for other people?
- What are the additional costs to me? Will insurance cover the costs?
- What is expected of me in terms of the amount of time or other involvement? Will I have to travel far to receive treatment, or can I receive it at a medical center near me?
- What side effects might I expect from this treatment? How much physical discomfort can I expect?
- Who is conducting the study, and who approved it? (Look for studies conducted by the National Institutes of Health, or by large hospitals or academic medical centers.)
- Can I get out of the trial whenever I want? (The answer should always be *yes*.)

Finding a Clinical Trial

Just because you want to participate in a clinical trial doesn't mean that one will necessarily be available to you. You may not "make the cut" for a variety of reasons.

"Good trials, as broad as they are in their eligibility, are actually quite narrow from the perspective of the population of patients who would potentially want to participate," says Maurie Markman, M.D., director of the Cleveland Clinic Taussig Cancer Center in Ohio. The type of people who can participate in a trial may be limited by the design of the experiment. For example, the study may admit only patients of a certain age or at a particular stage of disease or who have not already had certain other treatments. And since clinical trials can treat only a predetermined number of patients, the potential slots may fill quickly. Some fill their quota of participants through a lottery system.

The best way to find good clinical trials, conducted by reputable institutions and for which you are qualified to participate, is to talk with your doctor. A good doctor will work with you to locate an appropriate clinical trial in your area. He or she can more easily decipher the medical jargon that explains what is being studied in the trial and can determine your eligibility based on your medical history.

"Finding a good doctor is the most important thing," says Dr. Markman. "Wearing a white coat doesn't make me smarter or a better person, but it does give me a certain amount of knowledge. If you've got a complicated situation relative to your disease— you've got a bad heart, you've got a neurological condition, you've got diabetes—all these things will potentially influence [the decision to participate]. Your doctor knows all this. . . . Make sure you have a doctor you can trust who is willing to give you the information about what he or she knows, or will be in a position to gather information about trials that may be available to you either locally or regionally."

For more information about clinical trials, or to look up information about specific studies, go to www.clinicaltrials.gov on the Internet. This database, launched in February 2000 by the National Institutes of Health, provides information on more than 4,000 federal and private clinical trials at more than 47,000 locations in the United States. You can search the database by disease or by institution to get an idea of the kinds of research being conducted.

17. Final Notes

IF you've been diagnosed with a chronic illness or condition, finding information and making a preliminary treatment decision is just the beginning of a long process of improving and maintaining your health. Just as life itself is a continual process of change, your life will change because of your illness.

Although illness is never wished for or welcomed, it is possible to live a happy, fulfilled life in spite of disease. Even people with life-threatening conditions have found ways to turn their tragedy into an opportunity to live the type of life they always dreamed of, abandoning worry or concern for future problems, quitting a hated job, moving to a new house, taking a long-awaited trip, reconnecting to their spiritual selves, or simply speaking their minds freely for the first time in their lives. As Lillie Shockney, R.N., B.S., M.A.S., director of education and outreach at the Johns Hopkins Breast Center likes to say, "After diagnosis . . . you need to find your new 'normal,' which can be better than your old 'normal.'" Doctors, health professionals, family, friends, and other people with your disease can all help point you in a positive direction, but in the end, only you can determine how you react.

If you need more encouragement than that, here are a few more points to ponder:

• *About predicting the future:* "There is always a tremendous spectrum of each disease," says William C. Dooley, M.D., director of the Johns Hopkins Breast Center, "some much more rapid than others, and some much slower than you ever would have expected them to be. That's why it's easy to say what would happen with a thousand patients who look like this, but it's very difficult to say what would happen with a single patient." No one can predict the future, not even doctors. Don't let pronouncements about how much "time you have left" rule your life or your thoughts. Put your life in order, then live the life you have for however long it may be. "Don't just count the days . . . make each day count," says Lillie Shockney.

• *About creating priorities:* Serious illnesses have a way of pushing your dreams to the forefront of your life. Use that impetus to create the life you want. "I know I would not be where I am today, physically, mentally, or emotionally, if I hadn't had breast cancer," says Loretta, who survived a horrible surgical ordeal for breast cancer before finding good treatment. "You can't come across a life-threatening illness and come away without some purer sense of what you're supposed to be doing with your life, what the priorities in your life are, and how to take care of yourself."

• *About disease statistics:* Doctors use statistics to make educated guesses about the course of a disease or the side effects that might occur as the result of a treatment. They look at the odds and predict chances, but they can never say anything will happen for certain because statistics are based on groups of people, not on individuals. More than one oncologist has said that for any type of cancer, at any stage, someone in the world has had the disease and gone into remission—despite the odds, and for reasons no one understands. It's important to know where the "guesses" are coming from, but then understand that it is just a guess. It's also important to understand that statistics change. With each new study, each new treatment, each new medication, the factors that went into creating the statistics change. Keep looking for new information about your disease.

• *About the fear of making a decision:* When different treatment possibilities are suggested, choose the one that feels best for you. You won't be asked to make a decision you can't handle. "What I tell patients," says Susan Love, M.D., director of the nonprofit Susan Love Breast Cancer Foundation, "is that it's sort of like trying to decide whether to drive home on the scenic route or the freeway—you'll get there either way." She adds, "It's like any of these decisions we make in life, what college to go to, where to buy a house. . . . It ends up being a gut feeling."

• *About doing something:* Not all diagnoses require action. If you do enough testing, you're bound to find some disease in just about everyone. That doesn't mean that it is going to affect your life. For example, because of better technology and new blood tests, the probability of finding prostate cancer has increased in recent years. Prostate cancer incidence hasn't necessarily increased, but the *detection* of prostate cancer has. "So the difficulty is that then we will be detecting problems which will never be clinical problems during that person's lifetime," says Robert M. Kaplan, Ph.D., professor and chair of the Department of Family and Preventive Medicine at the University of California, San Diego. "In fact, according to autopsy studies, prostate cancer is quite common in older men. If a man gets a *diagnosis* of prostate cancer, it is likely that he'll be led down a path where he'll get surgical or radiation treatment for that condition. And it's quite likely that that treatment will make him impotent and/or incontinent, so there are quality of life consequences of treatment. For the great majority of those men who get treatment, they would never have known they had the disease during their lifetimes—that is, they never would have had symptoms, or had their life expectancies shortened because of the disease. So the consequences of, really, even looking for the disease may be even more severe than the condition itself."

So don't rush into action just because a particular test or treatment is available. Do the research, talk with your doctor, and find out whether you are really likely to be helped by doing something, versus doing nothing (often called "watchful waiting" by doctors).

• *About medical science:* Despite what we like to think, medicine is not perfect. It does not yet have all the answers, it cannot diagnose every disease, it cannot cure every disease, and the cures it offers may not always work. We can (and should) expect to be treated professionally, courteously, and with all the skill and technology afforded by the current state of medical knowledge, but we cannot expect perfection. At the same time, it is the best system we have for treating illness. Do not abandon medical science for an even less perfect mode of treatment.

• *About hope:* Many doctors generally prefer to treat patients who are realistic but hopeful. Unrealistic patients may overestimate their chances for survival and perhaps forgo treatments or avoid planning for future outcomes. Pessimistic patients can be difficult to treat because they come to the office with a "why bother" attitude. They are likely to stop taking medications, miss appointments, or give up entirely.

The concepts of optimism and hopefulness have been observed to be so important to a patient's well-being that some scientists have begun studying the benefits of a positive attitude in illness. Some studies have shown that people who are generally pessimistic—that is, having a negative outlook on life—have poorer physical health, are prone to depression, and have a higher rate of death than optimists—those who have a positive outlook on life. No one knows why this health difference happens, but it is possible that pessimists could be trained to change the way they think about life and life events, and thereby lower their risk of illness and death.

Don't let anyone take away your right to be hopeful. If your doctor gives up on you, find another doctor. If a friend or family member insists on dwelling on the negative side of your illness, ask them to stop talking that way in front of you.

• *About peace of mind:* There is the saying: "If you've got your health, you've got just about everything." Well, if you don't have your health, peace of mind is the next best thing. In health matters, peace of mind can come from searching out information about your illness, finding the right doctor, participating in treatment decisions, and knowing that you've done everything possible to take control of your health. That's the best any of us can do.

Selected References

Introduction

Association of American Medical Colleges Matriculating Student Questionnaire 1998: All Schools Report. AAMC, 1999.

FDA. CDER 1998 Report to the Nation: Improving Public Health Through Human Drugs. www.fda.gov.

Grumbach, K. Primary Care in the United States—The Best of Times, the Worst of Times. *NEJM*. December 23, 1999; 341(26):2008–2010.

Humayun, M. S., and E. deJuan, Jr. Artificial vision. *Eye*. 1998; 12 (pt 3b):605–607.

National Academies/Institute of Medicine Press Release. "Preventing Death and Injury from Medical Errors Requires Dramatic, System-Wide Changes." November 29, 1999. http://www4.national academies.org.

NIH. Cancer Death Rate Declined in the 1990s for the First Time Ever. http://cancernet.nci.nih.gov, December 16, 1999.

St. Peter, R. F., et al. Changes in the scope of care provided by primary care physicians. *NEJM*. December 23, 1999; 341(26):1980–1985.

Stafford, R. S., et al. Trends in adult visits to primary care physicians in the United States. *Arch Family Med*, January–February 1999; 8(1):26–32.

Zyzanski, S. J., et al. Trade-offs in high-volume primary care practice. *J Family Practice.* May 1998; 46(5):397–402.

1. Information—Why Bother?

Akabayashi, A., et al. Family consent, communication, and advance directives for cancer disclosure: A Japanese case and discussion. *J Med Ethics.* August 1999; 25(4):296–301.

American College of Physicians Ethics manual. Fourth edition. *Ann Intern Med.* April 1, 1998; 128(7):576–594.

Andersen, M. R., and N. Urban. Involvement in decision-making and breast cancer survivor quality of life. *Ann Behav Med.* Summer 1999; 21(3):201–209.

Balint, J., and W. Shelton. Regaining the initiative: Forging a new model of the patient-physician relationship. *JAMA.* March 20,1996; 275(11):887–891.

Barry, M. J. Involving patients in medical decisions: How can physicians do better? *JAMA.* December 22/29, 1999; 282(24):2356–2357.

Benbassat, J., et al. Patient's preferences for participation in clinical decision making: A review of published surveys. *Behavioral Medicine.* Summer 1998; 24:81–88.

Blanchard, C. G., et al. Information and decision-making preferences of hospitalized adult cancer patients. *Social Science Medicine.* 1988; 27(11):1139–1145.

Braddock, C. H., et al. Informed decision making in outpatient practice. *JAMA.* December 22/29, 1999; 282(24):2313–2320.

Charles, C., et al. Shared decision-making in the medical encounter: What does it mean? (Or, it takes at least two to tango). *Social Science Medicine.* 1997; 44(5):681–692.

Charles, C., et al. What do we mean by partnership in making decisions about treatment. *British Medical Journal.* September 18,1999; 319:780–782.

Elwyn, T, S., et al. Cancer disclosure in Japan: Historical comparisons, current practices. *Social Science Medicine.* May 1998; 46(9):1151–1163.

Frosch, D. L., and R. M. Kaplan. Shared decision making in clinical medicine: Past research and future directions. *Am J of Preventive Med.* 1999; 17(4):285–294.

Guadagnoli, E., P. Ward. Patient participation in decision-making. *Social Science Medicine.*1998; 47(3):329–339.

Hamadeh, G. N., and S. M. Adib. Cancer truth disclosure by Lebanese doctors. *Social Science Medicine.* November 1998; 47(9):1289–1294.

Jones, R., et al. Cross sectional survey of patients' satisfaction with information about cancer. *British Medical Journal.* November 6,1999; 319:1247–1248.

Kaplan, S. H., et al. Assessing the effects of physician-patient interactions on the outcomes of chronic disease. *Medical Care.* March 1989; 27(3 Supp):S110–S127.

Lang, F. The evolving roles of patient and physician. *Arch Fam Med.* January 2000; 9(1):65–67.

Lazovich, D., et al. Breast conservation therapy in the US following the 1990 NIH consensus development conference . . . *Cancer.* August 15, 1999; 86:628–637.

LeBlang, T. R. Informed consent and disclosure in the physician-patient relationship: Expanding obligations for physicians in the United States. *Medical Law.* 1995; 14(5–6):429–444.

Leflar, R. B. The cautious acceptance of informed consent in Japan. *Med Law.* 1997; 16(4):705–720.

Mahler, H. I., and J. A. Kulik. Effects of preparatory videotapes on self-efficacy beliefs and recovery from coronary bypass surgery. *Annals Behav Med.* Winter 1998; 20(1):39–46.

———. Preference for health care involvement, perceived control and surgical recovery: a prospective study. *Social Science Medicine.* 1990; 31(7):743–751.

Mitchell, J. L. Cross-cultural issues in the disclosure of cancer. *Cancer Practice.* May-June 1998; 6(3):153–160.

Nayfield, S. G., et al. Statutory requirements for disclosure of breast cancer treatment alternatives. *J National Cancer Institute.* August 17,1994; 86(16):1202–1208.

Ong, L. M. L., et al. Doctor-patient communication: A review of the literature. *Social Science Medicine.* 1995; 40(7):903–918.

Pierce, P. F. When the patient chooses: Describing unaided decisions in health care. *Human Factors.* 1996; 38(2):278–287.

Ross, S. D., et al. Clinical outcomes in statin treatment trials: A meta-analysis. *Archives of Internal Medicine.* August 9/23 1999; 159:1793–1802.

Staff: Journal of the National Cancer Institute. To Tell the truth: A cancer diagnosis in other cultures is often a family affair. *J Nat Can Inst.* November 17, 1999; 91(22):1918–1919.

Stewart, M. A. What is a successful doctor-patient interview? A study of interactions and outcomes. *Social Science Medicine.* 1984; 19(2):167–175.

Street, R. L., et al. Provider-patient communication and metabolic control. *Diabetes Care.* May 1993; 16(5):714–721.

Street, R. L., and B. Voigt. Patient participation in deciding breast cancer treatment and subsequent quality of life. *Medical Decision Making.* July–September 1997; 17(3):298–306.

Viinamaki, H., et al. The Patient-doctor relationship and metabolic control in patients with type 1 diabetes mellitus. *Intern. J of Psychiatry Med.* 1993; 23(3):265–274.

Vuori, H. Patient satisfaction—does it matter? *Qual Assur Health Care.* 1991; 3(3):183–189.

White, R., et al. Mood, learned resourcefulness and perceptions of control in type 1 diabetes mellitus. *J Psychosomatic Research.* February 1996; 40(2):205–212.

2. Becoming an Active Patient

Barry, M. J. Involving patients in medical decisions: How can physicians do better? *JAMA.* December 22/29, 1999; 282(24):2356–2357.

Braddock, C. H., III; K. A. Edwards; et al. Informed decision making in outpatient practice: Time to get back to basics. *JAMA.* December 22/29, 1999; 282(24):2313–2320.

Bruera, E.; E. Pituskin; et al. The Addition of an audiocassette recording of a consultation to written recommendations for patients with advanced cancer: A randomized, controlled trial. *Cancer.* December 1999; 86(11):2420–2425.

Cegala, D. J. Communicating with your doctor. Private publication, 1997.

Cegala, D. J.; T. Marinelli; and D. Post. The Effects of patient communication skills training on compliance. *Arch Fam Med.* January 2000; 9(1):57–64.

Cegala, D. J.; L. McClure; T. M. Marinelli; and D. M. Post. The Effects of communication skills training on patients' participation during medical interviews. *Patient Ed & Counseling.* In press.

Johnson, I. A., and D. J. Adelstein. The Use of recorded interviews to enhance physician-patient communication. *J Cancer Educ.* 1991; 6(2):99–102.

Labrecque, M. S.; C. G. Blanchard; et al. The Impact of family presence on the physician–cancer patient interaction. *Soc Sci Med*. 1991; 33(11):1253–1261.

Lang, F. The Evolving roles of patient and physician. *Arch Fam Med*. January 2000; 9(1):65–67.

Tattersall, M. H.; P. N. Butow; et al. The Take-home message: patients prefer consultation audiotapes to summary letters. *J Clin Oncol*. June 1994; 12(6):1305–1311.

6. Mass Media: Newspapers, Television, Radio

Frucht, S.; J. D. Rogers; et al Falling asleep at the wheel: Motor vehicle mishaps in persons taking pramipexole and ropinirole. *Neurology*. June 10, 1999; 52(9):1908–1910.

Fuchs, C. S.; E. L. Giovannucci; et al. Dietary fiber and the risk of colorectal cancer and adenoma in women. *NEJM*. January 21, 1999; 340(3):169–176.

Hackman, E. M., and G. L. Moe. Evaluation of newspaper reports of nutrition-related research. *J Am Dietetic Assn*. December 1999; 99(12):1564–1566.

Hu, F. B.; M. J. Stampfer; et al. A Prospective study of egg consumption and risk of cardiovascular disease in men and women. *JAMA*. April 21,1999; 281(15):1387–1394.

Iribarren, C., et al. Effect of cigar smoking on the risk of cardiovascular disease, chronic obstructive pulmonary disease, and cancer in men. *NEJM*. June 10, 1999; 340(23):1773–1780.

Okumura, K.; K. Iseki; et al. Low serum cholesterol as a risk factor for hemorrhagic stroke in men: A community-based mass screening in Okinawa, Japan. *Jpn Circ J*. January 1999; 63(1):53–58.

Potter, J. D. Fiber and colorectal cancer—where to now? *NEJM*. January 21,1999; 340(3):223–224.

Powell, N. B.; R. W. Riley; and C. Guilleminault. Radiofrequency tongue base reduction in sleep-disordered breathing: A pilot study. *Otolaryngol Head Neck Surg*. May 1999; 120(5):656–664.

8. Internet

Gagel, M. P. The Internet—a new information medium for nurses, part 2. *Canadian Onc Nursing J*. 1999; 9(1):3–9.

Jadad, A. R.; R. B. Haynes; et al. The Internet and evidence-based decision-making: A needed synergy for efficient knowledge management in health care. *CMAJ.* 2000; 162(3):362–365.

Markman, M. Cancer information and the Internet: Benefits and risks. *Cleveland Clinic J of Med.* May 1998; 65(5):274–276.

Mehta, N. Searching the Internet for medical information: Practical tips. *Cleveland Clinic J of Med.* October 1999; 66(9):543–546, 549–550, 553.

Pandolfini, C.; P. Impicciatore; and M. Bonati. Parents on the Web: Risks for quality management of cough in children. *Pediatrics.* January 2000; 105(1):e1. www.pediatrics.org.

White, H.; E. McConnell; et al. Surfing the Net in later life: A review of the literature and pilot study of computer use and quality of life. *J Appl Gerontology.* September 1999; 18(3):358–378.

Winker, M. A.; A. Flanagin; et al. Guidelines for medical and health information sites on the Internet. *JAMA.* March 22/29, 2000; 283(12):1600–1606.

9. Medical Journals and MEDLINE

Greenhalgh, T. How to read a paper: Getting your bearings (deciding what the paper is about). *BMJ.* July 26, 1997; 315:243–246.

Pitkin, R. M.; M. A. Branagan; and L. F. Burmeister. Accuracy of data in abstracts of published research articles. *JAMA.* March 24/31, 1999; 281(12):1110–1111.

11. Doctors

Bagenstose, S. E., and J. A. Bernstein. Treatment of chronic rhinitis by an allergy specialist improves quality of life outcomes. *Ann Allergy Asthma Immunol.* December 1999; 83(6Pt1):524–528.

Bello, D.; N. B. Shah; et al. Self-reported differences between cardiologists and heart failure specialists in the management of chronic heart failure. *Am Heart J.* July 1999; 138(1Pt1):100–107.

Bindman, A. B. Can physician profiles be trusted? *JAMA* (editorial). June 1999; 281(22):2142–2143.

Casale, P. N., et al. Patients treated by cardiologists have a lower in-hospital mortality for acute myocardial infarction. *J Am Coll Cardiol.* October 1998; 32(4):885–889.

Gums, J. G., et al. A Randomized, prospective study measuring outcomes after antibiotic therapy intervention by a multidisciplinary consult team. *Pharmacotherapy*. December 1999; 19(12):1369–1377.

Harrold, L. R.; T. S. Field; and J. H. Gurwitz. Knowledge, patterns of care, and outcomes of care for generalists and specialists. *J Gen Internal Med*. August 1999; 14(8):499–511.

Hofer, T. P., et al. The Unreliability of individual physician "report cards" for assessing the costs and quality of care of a chronic disease. *JAMA*. June 1999; 281(22):2098–2105.

Jollis, J. G.; E. R. DeLong; et al. Outcome of acute myocardial infarction according to the specialty of the admitting physician. *NEJM*. December 19, 1996; 335(25):1880–1887.

Levetan, C. S., et al. Effect of physician specialty on outcomes in diabetic ketoacidosis. *Diabetes Care*. November 1999; 22(11):1790–1795.

Meagher, A. P. Colorectal cancer: Is the surgeon a prognostic factor? A systematic review. *Med J Aust*. September 20, 1999; 171(6):308–310.

Morrison, J., and P. Wickersham. Physicians disciplined by a state medical board. *JAMA*. June 1998; 279(23):1889–1893.

Nash, I. S.; R. R. Corrato; et al. Generalist versus specialist care for acute myocardial infarction. *Am J Cardiol*. March 1, 1999; 83(5):650–654.

Vickrey, B. G.; Z. V. Edmonds; et al. General neurologist and subspecialist care for multiple sclerosis: Patient's perceptions. *Neurology*. Oct 12, 1999; 53(6):1190–1197.

12. Hospitals

Ayanian, J. Z.; J. S. Weissman; et al. Quality of care for two common illnesses in teaching and nonteaching hospitals. *Health Aff (Millwood)*. November–December 1998; 17(6):194–205.

Bentley, J. M., and D. B. Nash. How Pennsylvania hospitals have responded to publicly released reports on coronary artery bypass graft surgery. *Jt Comm J Qual Improv*. January 1998; 24(1):40–49.

Birkmeyer, J. D. High-risk surgery—follow the crowd. *JAMA*. March 1, 2000; 283(9):1191–1193.

Dudley, R. A.; K. L. Johansen; et al. Selective referral to high-volume hospitals: Estimating potentially avoidable deaths. *JAMA*. March 1, 2000; 283(9):1159–1166.

Epstein, A. M. Public release of performance data: A progress report from the front. *JAMA*. April 12, 2000; 283(14):1884–1886.

————. Rolling down the runway: The challenges ahead for quality report cards. *JAMA*. June 3, 1998; 279(21):1691–1696.

Frost, M. H.; R. D. Arvizu; et al. A Multidisciplinary healthcare delivery model for women with breast cancer: Patient satisfaction and physical and psychosocial adjustment. *Oncol Nurs Forum*. November–December 1999; 26(10):1673–1680.

Gabel, M.; N. E. Hilton; and S. D. Nathanson. Multidisciplinary breast cancer clinics. Do they work? *Cancer*. June 15, 1997; 79(12):2380–2384.

Hall, R. E., and M. M. Cohen. Variations in hysterectomy rates in Ontario: Does the indication matter? *CMAJ*. December 15, 1994; 151(12):1713–1719.

Hill, C. A.; K. L. Winfrey; and B. A. Rudolph. "Best hospitals": A Description of the methodology for the index of hospital quality. *Inquiry*. Spring 1997; 34(1):80–90.

Hofer, T. P., and R. A. Hayward. Identifying poor-quality hospitals. Can hospital mortality rates detect quality problems for medical diagnoses? *Med Care*. August 1996; 34(8):737–753.

Jollis, J. G.; E. D. Peterson; et al. Relationship between physician and hospital coronary angioplasty volume and outcome in elderly patients. *Circulation*. June 3, 1997; 95(11):2485–2491.

Longo, D. R.; G. Land; et al. Consumer reports in health care. Do they make a difference in patient care? *JAMA*. November 19, 1997; 278(19):1579–1584.

Marshall, M. N.; P. G. Shekelle; et al. The public release of performance data: What do we expect to gain? A review of the evidence. *JAMA*. April 12, 2000; 283(14):1866–1874.

Mennemeyer, S. T.; M. A. Morrisey; and L. Z. Howard. Death and reputation: How consumers acted upon HCFA mortality information. *Inquiry*. Summer 1997; 34(2):117–128.

O'Connor, G. T.; S. K. Plume; et al. A regional intervention to improve the hospital mortality associated with coronary artery bypass graft surgery. The northern New England cardiovascular disease study group. *JAMA*. March 20, 1996; 275(11):841–846.

Rosenthal, G. E.; M. M. Chren; R. J. Lasek; and C. S. Landefeld. What patients should ask of consumers' guides to health care quality. *Eval Health Professions*. September 1998; 21(3):316–331.

Rosenthal, G. E.; D. L. Harper; L. M. Quinn; and G. S. Cooper. Severity-adjusted mortality and length of stay in teaching and nonteaching hospitals. Results of a regional study. *JAMA*. August 13, 1997; 278(6):485–490.

Rosenthal, G. E.; L. Quinn; and D. L. Harper. Declines in hospital mortality associated with a regional initiative to measure hospital performance. *Am J Med Qual*. Summer 1997; 12(2):103–112.

Rosenthal, G. E.; A. Shah; L. E. Way; and D. L. Harper. Variations in standardized hospital mortality rates for six common medical diagnoses: Implications for profiling hospital quality. *Med Care*. July 1998; 36(7):955–964.

Yao, S. L., and G. Lu-Yao. Population-based study of relationships between hospital volume of prostatectomies, patient outcomes, and length of hospital stay. *J Nat Cancer Inst*. November 17, 1999; 91(22):1950–1956.

13. Complementary Medicine or Self-Care

Barrett, S., and V. Herbert. More ploys that may fool you. *http://www.quackwatch.com/01QuackeryRelatedTopics/ploys.html*.

Boullata, J. I., and A. M. Nace. Safety issues with herbal medicine. *Pharmacotherapy*. March 2000; 20(3):257–269.

Cassileth, B. R. Complementary and alternative cancer medicine. *Journal of Clinical Oncology*. November 1999; 17(11 suppl.):44–52.

———. Complementary therapies: The American experience. *Supportive Care in Cancer*. January 2000; 8(1):16–23.

Gaster, B., and J. Holroyd. St. John's wort for depression: A systematic review. *Archives of Internal Medicine*. January 24, 2000; 160(2):152–156.

Hirata, J. D.; L. M. Swiersz; et al. Does dong quai have estrogenic effects in postmenopausal women? A double-blind, placebo-controlled trial. *Fertility and Sterility*. December 1997; 68(6):981–986.

Jacobson, J. S.; S. B. Workman; and F. Kronenberg. Research on complementary/alternative medicine for patients with breast cancer: A review of biomedical literature. *Journal of Clinical Oncology*. February 2000; 18(3):668–683.

Jarvis, W. T. Quackery: The National Council Against Health Fraud perspective. *Rheum Dis Clin North Am*. November 1999; 25(4):805–814.

Kessler, D. A. Editorial: Cancer and herbs. *New England Journal of Medicine*. June 8, 2000; 342(23):1742–1743.

Lis-Balchin, M. Possible health and safety problems in the use of novel plant essential oils and extracts in aromatherapy. *Journal of the Royal Society of Health*. December 1999; 119(4):240–243.

Metz, J. M. Personal communication of study results presented at the American Society of Clinical Oncology meeting, May 2000.

Ness, J.; F. T. Sherman; and C. X. Pan. Alternative medicine: What the data say about common herbal therapies. *Geriatrics*. October 1999; 54(10):33–38, 40, 43.

Nortier, J. L., et al. Urothelial carcinoma associated with the use of a Chinese herb (Aristolochia fangchi). *New England Journal of Medicine*. June 8, 2000; 342(23):1686–1692.

Special article—Is integrative medicine the medicine of the future: A debate between Arnold S. Relman, M.D., and Andrew Weil, M.D. *Archives of Internal Medicine*. Oct 11, 1999; 159(18):2122–2126.

Verhoef, M. J.; R. J. Hilsden; and M. O'Beirne. Complementary therapies and cancer care: An overview. *Patient Education & Counseling*. October 1999; 38(2):93–100.

Zink, T., and J. Chaffin. Herbal "health" products: What family physicians need to know. *American Family Physician*. October 1, 1998; 58(5):1133–1140.

14. Other Caregivers

Alberts, M. S., et al. Psychological interventions in the pre-surgical period. *Int J Psychiatry Med*. 1989; 19(1):91–106.

Bloom, B. S., and R. C. Iannacone. Internet availability of prescription pharmaceuticals to the public. *Annals Internal Med*. December 7, 1999; 131(11):830–833.

Cunningham, A. J.; C. V. I. Edmonds; et al. A Randomized controlled trial of the effects of group psychological therapy on survival in women with breast cancer. *Psycho-Oncology*. 1998; 7:508–517.

Galinsky, M. J., and J. H. Schopler. Negative experiences in support groups. *Social Work in Health Care*. 1994; 20(1):77–95.

Helgeson, V. S.; S. Cohen; et al. Education and peer discussion group interventions and adjustment to breast cancer. *Arch Gen Psychiatry*. April 1999; 56:340–347.

Helgeson, V. S.; S. Cohen; et al. Group support interventions for women with breast cancer: Who benefits from what? *Health Psychology*. 2000; 19(2):107–114.

Henney, J. E.; J. E. Shuren; et al. Internet purchase of prescription drugs: Buyer beware. *Annals Internal Med*. December 7, 1999; 131(11): 861–862.

Mumford, E.; H. J. Schlesinger; and G. V. Glass. The Effect of psychological intervention on recovery from surgery and heart attacks: An analysis of the literature. *Am J Public Health*. February 1982; 72(2):141–151.

Schopler, J. H., and M. J. Galinsky. Support groups as open systems: A model for practice and research. *Health and Social Work*. 1993; 18(3):195–207.

Spiegel, D.; J. R. Bloom; H. C. Kraemer; and E. Gottheil. Effect of psychosocial treatment on survival of patients with metastatic breast cancer. *Lancet*. October 14,1989; 2(8668):888–891.

West, D. S. On-line pharmacies: Implications for the future. *Drug Topics*. May 1, 2000:83–90.

16. Shared Decision Making

Barry, M. J.; F. J. Fowler; et al. Patient reactions to a program designed to facilitate patient participation in treatment decisions for benign prostatic hyperplasia. *Med Care*. 1995; 33(8):771–782.

Charles, C.; A. Gafni; and T. Whelan. Decision-making in the physician-patient encounter: Revisiting the shared treatment decision-making model. *Soc Sic Med*. 1999; 49:651–661.

Deber, R. B. Shared decision making in the real world. *J Gen Intern Med*. June 1996; 11(6):377–378.

Deber, R. B.; N. Kraetschmer; and J. Irvine. What role do patients wish to play in treatment decision making? *Arch Intern Med*. July 8, 1996; 156(13):1414–1420.

Erlen, J. A. Treatment decision making: Who should decide? *Orthopaedic Nursing*. July–August 1998; 17(4):60–64.

Frosch, D. L., and R. M. Kaplan. Shared decision making in clinical medicine: Past research and future directions. *Am J of Preventive Med*. 1999; 17(4):285–294.

Gafni, A.; C. Charles; and T. Whelan. The physician-patient encounter: The physician as a perfect agent for the patient versus the informed treatment decision-making model. *Soc Sci Med*. 1998; 47(3):347–354.

Guadagnoli, E.; and P. Ward. Patient participation in decision-making. *Soc Sci Med*. 1998; 47(3):329–339.

Kaplan, R. M. Health-related quality of life in patient decision making. *J of Social Issues.* 1991; 47(4):69–90.

———. An Outcomes-based model for directing decisions in women's health care. *Clin Obstet Gynecol.* March 1994; 37(1):192–206.

———. Shared medical decision-making: A new paradigm for behavioral medicine—1997 Presidential Address. Society of Behavioral Medicine, San Francisco, California. April 1997.

Liao, L.; J. G. Jollis; et al. Impact of an interactive video on decision making of patients with ischemic heart disease. *J Gen Intern Med.* 1996; 11:373–376.

Markman, M. Why should cancer patients participate in clinical trials? *Cleveland Clinic J of Med.* October 1998; 65(9):497–499.

Mazur, D. J. *Shared Decision Making in the Patient-Physican Relationship: Challenges for Patients, Physicians, and Medical Institutions.* Tampa, FL: American College of Physician Executives, 2000.

Mazur, D. J.; and D. H. Hickam. Patients' preferences for risk disclosure and role in decision making for invasive medical procedures. *J Gen Intern Med.* 1997; 12:114–117.

Mazur, D. J.; D. H. Hickam; and M. D. Mazur. How patients' preferences for risk information influence treatment choice in a case of high risk and high therapeutic uncertainty: Asymptomatic localized prostate cancer. *Med Decis Making.* 1999; 19:394–398.

Mazur, D. J., and J. F. Merz. Patients' interpretations of verbal expressions of probability: Implications for securing informed consent to medical interventions. *Behav Sci Law.* Autumn 1994; 12(4):417–426.

Mort, E. A. Clincial decision-making in the face of scientific uncertainty: Hormone replacement therapy as an example. *J Fam Pract.* 1996; l42:147–151.

O'Connor, A. M.; A. Rostom; et al. Decision aids for patients facing health treatment or screening decisions: A Systematic review. *British Medical Journal.* September 18, 1999; 319:731–734.

O'Connor, A. M.; P. Tugwell; et al. A Decision aid for women considering hormone therapy after menopause: Decision support framework and evaluation. *Patient Educ Couns.* March 1998; 33(3):267–279.

Onel, E.; C. Hamond; et al. Assessment of the feasibility and impact of shared decision making in prostate cancer. *Urology.* 1998; 51:63–66.

Patel, S. C., and G. L. Spaeth. Compliance in patients prescribed eyedrops for glaucoma. *Ophthalmic Surg.* May–June 1995; 26(3):233–236.

Piercy, G. B.; R. Deber; et al. Impact of a shared decision-making program on patients with benign prostatic hyperplasia. *Urology.* 1999; 53:913–920.

Whelan, T.; M. Levine; et al. Mastectomy or lumpectomy? Helping women make informed choices. *J Clin Oncol.* June 1999; 17(6):1727–1735.

17. Final Notes

Maruta, T.; R. C. Colligan; et al. Optimists vs. pessimists: Survival rate among medical patients over a 30-year period. *Mayo Clin Proc.* 2000; 75:140–143.

Peterson, C.; M. E. Seligman; G. E. Vaillant. Pessimistic explanatory style is a risk factor for physical illness: A thirty-five-year longitudinal study. *J Pers Soc Psychol.*1988; 55:23–27.

Seligman, M. E.; L. Y. Abramson; et al. Depressive attributional style. *J Abnorm Psychol.* 1979; 88:242–247.

Index